UNDRESSED

Deborah Kagan

UNDRESSED

An Invitation to Claim Your Erotic Nature

Urano
publishing

Argentina - Chile - Colombia - Spain
USA - Mexico - Peru - Uruguay

© 2023 by Urano Publishing, an imprint of Urano World USA, Inc

8871 SW 129th Terrace Miami FL 33176 USA

Urano
publishing

Cover art and design by Sandra de Waard

Cover copyright © Urano Publishing, an imprint of Urano World USA, Inc

The first edition of this book was published in October 2023

ISBN: 978-1-953027-18-4

E-ISBN: 978-1-953027-21-4

Printed in Spain

Library of Cataloging-in-Publication Data

Kagan, Deborah

1. Feminism   2. Spirituality & Sexuality

Undressed: An Invitation to Claim Your Erotic Nature

Praise For Undressed

"This book is charged with the kind of energy that inspires women to think differently about what they are allowed to claim as their pleasure.

I am so grateful to Deborah for her commitment to her sacred quest into healing from loss and sexual trauma that unfortunately so many women also deal with. Deborah delivers real juicy sex talk straight from her very own body wisdom. She so generously shares her erotic life with us so that we can learn what unabashed desire to fully meet everything life has to offer can look like for women.

You will become besotted with each chapter and its thrilling and emotional eroticas, that also offers the reader a kinky self love practice to tap into your own sacred eros. May you find this book as a companion so you don't have to walk the path alone.

~ Rie Katagiri, Movement and Intimacy Coach, creator of Erotic Movement Arts

Deborah Kagan breaks radical new ground by undressing herself and you the reader in a naked, honest, no-holes-barred, throbbing, glistening manual of empowerment, self-loving and flowering into your sacred aliveness. Her mandala is unique, raw, and deeply alive. Leave hesitation and shame at the door and dive into this feast for your mind, senses, and soul. Are YOU experienced? When you fall into your baptism in the bliss, power and radiance that flows through you as you read, you absolutely will be! Very highly recommended.

—David Kennedy, awakening coach and author of *Feng Shui for Dummies* and *Feng Shui Tips for a Better Life*

"*Undressed* is a deeply empowering, hands on, step by step, luscious guide inviting us to reclaim our erotic nature. It's filled with sexy story-telling and inspiring exercises. Kagan is our fearless, funny, whip smart and totally trustable companion on a journey to deep pleasure, power and erotic possibility."

~ Heidi Rose Robbins, Author of *Everyday Radiance* and *Zodiac Love Letters*

This is an inspirational memoir that weaves sex, spirituality, consciousness, and courage. Ladies, get your highlighters out because there is so much amazing knowledge in this book you are going to want to revisit these concepts over and over.

Deborah's deeply honest and evocative style cracks open my own memories of past lovers. It has me pondering what I learned from the men with whom I have shared myself and maybe even them from me. Deborah gives us a mirror allowing us to feel seen, as I have had so many of the same fears, self-doubts, and heartbreaks which she so fearlessly shares. Then she gives us tools to help us break some of these beliefs and wounds.

Deborah has a way of making me laugh and cry with her as she courageously shares her most private life moments. She encourages us to look at ourselves, to discover our feminine power, and teaches us how to be more unabashedly Mojolicious®.

~ Angela Tortu, Director of TV (Netflix, ABC, NBC, CBS, Disney+, HBOMax, Paramount+) and Film

Too often we let our erotic nature go unexplored. "Undressed" is the invitation you need to claim and relish your sensual self. Part memoir, part how-to, and part meditation, Kagan's book joyously takes us on a sexy, liberating and fulsome journey to our own sexuality. Mojolicious® in every way!

~ Sarah Chadwick, Author of *The Sweetness of Venus: A History of the Clitoris*

For women seeking to go beyond, just connection to their own pleasure, and bust out into true extraordinary, erotic life experiences, this book is the roadmap with all the twists and turns expertly navigated. Deborah leads by example and walks you through processes to embrace your own innate sexuality. It combines erotic examples of a turned on woman's intriguingly sexual life experiences with ways to bring that sexy eroticism into your own life. This is a book that's meant to be savored.

~ Susan Bratton, Intimacy Expert to Millions

Many strong, wise, brave women on the planet right now are processing and rewriting the archetype of being 'burnt at the stake' for sharing their unapologetic bigness, standing in their erotic power, processing and reframing the traumatized ancestral lineage of exiled and imprisoned women.

The shadow of this is that some of these women have found themselves unconsciously exhausting themselves to keep 'pretty', to keep 'sexy', to keep 'being a caring Mother', to keep 'popular', to keep the peace and not risk exile and violence. I want to salute and support, Deborah Kagan and her book, *Undressed*. It is a call to dissolve that fake scaffolding and pull out the splinter of the internalized beliefs 'I am not to be erotic, I am not to be free, I am not to be exactly myself'. Thank you, Deborah for being a part of the army of permission we are all creating in the Quickening!

~Jamie Catto, Author, Filmmaker, and Musician

Author's Disclaimer

This work depicts actual events in my life as truthfully as recollection and detailed journal entries permit. All experiences were my choice—I am not advocating for or against them, merely offering them to you as a possible perspective. The practices and advice included are based on my personal and professional experience. Although I am a Mentor for women, if you are not an active, current client, I am not your Mentor and you should consult the appropriate professional with respect to your physical, emotional, or spiritual well-being. The publisher and I are not responsible for any adverse effects or consequences resulting from the use of any of the suggestions, preparations, or practices discussed in this book.

Please note: This book is intended for 18+ adult readers. It deals with explicit sex, including brief mentions of sexual assault and domestic violence. While, the topics are dealt with in a compassionate and respectful manner, I understand it might be troubling for some readers. Discretion is advised.

This book is about empowering yourself as a woman. To that end, I am a staunch advocate for safe, consensual sex—each and every time.

UNDRESSED

Also by Deborah Kagan

*Find Your ME Spot: Reclaim Your Confidence, Feel Good in
Your Own Skin and Live a Turned On Life*

UNDRESSED

An Invitation to Claim Your Erotic Nature

Deborah Kagan

for the Divine Feminine in us all

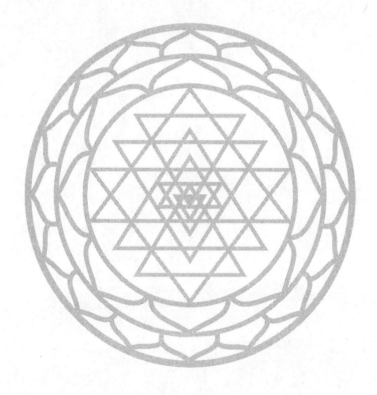

In honor of every woman's stolen pleasure, I reclaim it

You're healing my narrative of how I speak, treat, think, feel and embody my sexuality and practice with pleasure

It is my right to have gooey connection, God created sex and I am seeing sex as a sacred art the highest meditation, the most creative prayer

Breathing in and out, satisfactory presence, mind blowing intimacy is my blessing

This right here is pure, this is good, this is holy and again this is pure

~ Toni Jones, Lyrics from *Kiss Me*

TABLE OF CONTENTS

Section Five: Throat

Section Six: Third Eye

Section Seven: Crown

PREFACE

aka: Hello, Pussy

Greetings. This is your pussy speaking. I am relieved you're here. It's been a while. And let me say, your *hard to get game* is on pointe. Honestly, I wasn't sure we'd find each other again. But here's the thing, you and me—we're a team. For instance, you sit on me every day. I know we've been through some *stuff* over the years. What's important to remember is that I am here for you.

Always have been.

Now that we're reconnecting, let's clarify a few things.

I am yours. As in, when you take ownership of me it makes our partnership possible. It's nearly impossible to give you everything that's available here if you deny me and my existence. I don't need you to be hyperaware or thinking about me 24/7—but a daily check in would rock. Here's why. When you and I have a working, living, breathing relationship, I can offer you the world.

I know. I know. You're skeptical. So many people have tried to turn you against me over the years. Could be your parents, misinformed sex-ed, your religion, other women, and for sure, the patriarchy. That doesn't make them right. They are the ones afraid of what you and I can do together. They know that if you and I connect and form a real relationship *and* all the other humans with pussies do the same with theirs—well, there will be some serious overdue changes made. They like it the way it is. But *you're here*. And that means on some level, you are ready for change.

Hey. Deep breath. In and out.

I promise—connecting with me is not that scary.

The fact that you're here is a good sign. At the very least it means you are hearing my whispers, and maybe even my rants and shouts. Like when I tell you to hold off on the meeting with that colleague. The one that makes you nervous. And you reschedule to a day when your confidence is intact. Well done! Or when you desperately want to go to the super cool event you heard about from your friend. You think the invite won't show up and consider making plans with your family instead. Alas! You hear me nudging you to hold off. Whallah! The invite comes in!

I am just trying to get your attention because you and I are about to take this journey together.

I wrangled Deborah and her pussy to write this book (don't you love the idea that all pussies communicate covertly all the time, on all levels of existence... wink, wink). We got her to document the awakening and reclamation of *her* pussy and erotic nature. Now, before you get all twitchy about the word erotic, let me give you the simple definition:

1. of, devoted to, or tending to arouse sexual love or desire
2. strongly marked or affected by sexual desire.

I guess this is also a good time to distinguish what we mean by sexual desire.

Let's break it down. The world/universe/Gaia/cosmos is made up of energy. Those smart fuckers, physicists specifically, the quantum ones, thankfully got it together to prove to humans that *energy is real*. And every-friggin-thing is made up of it. You, me, stars, clothes, dildos, flowers, bees... you get the picture. All of this universal energy is what moves life forward. It's the cosmic thrust continuously seeking more of itself. Not unlike me when I glide into those multiple orgasm moments riding more and more and more and more... oh wait! I'm getting ahead of myself.

The point is—everything is energy. Some people call it chi or qi (usually those are the Feng Shui, Tai Chi, Qigong, martial arts folks). The Yogis call it prana. Some people call it life force (Pagans, Wiccans, or Eurocentric folks) and others call it sexual energy (usually those are the New Age, metaphysical folks). Some people call it Mojo (usually those are the urban centric ancestor sourced folks... and honestly, that's what Deborah and I like to call it). Whatever word you use for it, it is the energy that animates all life in all forms. It births more. All the time. Every day. And it doesn't discriminate.

The cool thing is you have a storehouse of this Mojo in you. It's located between your belly button and pubic bone. Spanning the whole space from the front of your body to the back. And guess what? I am the gateway to it. Well, technically the part of me called the cervix is the actual doorway, but we'll get to that later in the book. For now, it's critical to get that I am the access to your deepest and most profound levels of Mojo. Surprised? That's ok. I'm used to people shirking me off, shoving me down, deep between their thighs, and hoping to forget that I even exist!

So, getting back to sexual desire.

Sexual means: of or relating to sex or the sexes.

Desire means: to long or hope for, to express a wish for: request.

Let's look at sexual desire. Not exclusively related to the act of sex, but for what it more accurately is:

The mechanism with which you energetically beam out what it is you deeply want in life.

Pretty incredible, right?

Imagine this:

- The more rooted you are in your sexual desire, the more honestly you own your erotic nature.
- The more honestly you own your erotic nature, the closer you are to me, your pussy.
- The closer you are to me, the more alive, powerful, and confident you feel every day.
- The more alive, powerful, and confident you feel, the easier it is to create a life you actually want.
- The easier it is to create that life, the greater the contribution you become to everything and everyone around you.

And that, m'dear, is why I continue to holler at you and finally, get to clap our lips that you are here reading this book! You and me, baby. We can make anything happen.

Here's the other thing to know. Some things Deborah writes about might stir up *feelings*. She and her pussy did their best to bring you a wide range of them. My advice, and please start taking it because I'm the part of you tapped into your Universal Truth, is that you let yourself go on the ride of this book. There's no rush. You can pace it out. As long as you keep going and give yourself space to explore, expand, and get more rooted in our connection—we'll be golden.

Deborah's pussy intentionally calls this book UNDRESSED. There's the obvious reason that when you and I are at our most basic, we're naked. No clothes. The thing is that emotionally, psychologically, and spiritually, we acquired many layers of invisible clothing over the years. My job with you, and why I brought you to this book, is to take off these outdated layers that, at this point, only serve to hold us back.

I need you to undress as Deborah and her pussy invite you to do in the pages of this book.

There are helpful resources in every chapter and online support as well. Plus, Deborah and her pussy have a vibrant online community. I highly recommend you get involved with them to ask questions, meet other women saying hello to their pussies, and be in the empowering conversation Deborah and her pussy continue to hold space for year after year.

If you can feel a little tingle in me right now that's because I am beside myself, in the best way, that we're reconnecting. I love being with you. I love being yours. I know what's possible when you and I are an awakened, conscious team. And I am here for it!

OK. Enough from me for the moment.

Enjoy getting undressed with Deborah.

But please remember, pay attention to my whispers, shoves, and shouts as you take the journey.

Love + Mojo,

Your Pussy 💋

INTRODUCTION

Welcome! So happy to meet you

One of the only moments I remember from before the age of six is playing "doctor" with the little boy across the street. We both thought it a novel idea and agreed to assume the roles. I can still remember the flush of excitement. The rush of heat in a body that was too small to understand it. The innocent curiosity of being the examiner and then the patient. How it felt fun and free, like the midafternoon sun streaming in the window without a care in the world. And then, *then*, you can guess what happens next. The adults screaming. *What are you two doing?! NO! Don't ever do that again. You're not supposed to let that happen. What's wrong with you?* What was like the gleeful mystery of unwrapping holiday presents became an instant underground taboo. The freedom, pleasure, and joy dashed out the window leaving only their shadows (shame, despair, guilt, and psychospiritual restriction).

A flicker of the aliveness I felt that afternoon peeked its head up two years later. My Mom picked me up early from school. It was a Friday in 1978. I was seven. She took me to the Ziegfeld Theater in our home town of New York City on a ladies date. Carrying the popcorn and Milk Duds up to our seats in the balcony,

I felt grown up—and a little naughty skipping the last few hours of school. But we were there for an important movie. Everyone was talking about it—Grease. The lights went down, the screen lit up, and my little body came alive. John Travolta's good boy/bad boy lightning shot through my veins. Olivia Newton John's black shiny leggings and big hair transformation made me giggle and cheer. It was Stockard Channing's Rizzo that got under my skin. The tough chick. The provocative chick. The *loose* chick. I loved her Mojo. The way she had confidence, sass, and wasn't afraid to flaunt it. Even though I didn't understand the deeper meaning, my little heart hurt for her when she sang "There are Worse Things I Could Do." For months after seeing the film, I'd grab my hairbrush (aka microphone), pop in the eight track of the soundtrack, jump on my bed, and perform the entire story. It made me want to live. As if the adventures they sang of were possible for me too. Including all the vibrancy, freedom, and self-expression. It quieted my confused brain as my Mom started dating the man that was to become her second husband, and the domestic abuser we lived with for eight long years. His highly erratic emotional abuse was directed to both of us. Only in the last couple years of the marriage was the physical directed to me as well as my Mom. Growing up with that kind of chaos in the home, watching my Mom hide in my room to avoid him night after night, and having the authorities show up regularly instilled a feeling that women have no power. That they have no autonomy. And that their bodies are to be abused. Performing the soundtrack to Grease for most of my childhood gave me hope that I could become strong, confident, and sensually alive.

Thirty years later and a lot of life under my belt, I found myself walking into the Superdome Arena in New Orleans. The tenth anniversary of VDAY, a global organization to end violence to women and girls, was having a multiday event. Wearing a pink floor length ruffled skirt with white polka dots and a t-shirt with a cherubic kitten and the words, *Love Your Pussy*, under it, I bounced through the giant vulva decorated entrance. Two steps into the arena and what felt like a bolt of cosmic connection stopped me in my tracks. *Boing!* What the...? I stood frozen. Then, I heard it. What I like to call, *the shove from above*. Some people call it a god wink or the voice of your Higher Self. It pierced me with a very clear message. *Deborah*, it said emphatically, *it's time to get up off your ass and do the work with women.* Quietly, I replied, *OK. I'm not sure what you want me to do—AND I'm listening.*

After that trip, I returned home to Los Angeles and met up with a girlfriend at Urth Caffe. Green tea latte in hand, *The Shove* showed up and turned a switch on in my mind. I blurted out, *I got it! I'm going to start a women's group. It'll be a safe place to talk about our bodies, sex, intimate relating, spirituality, and being a juicy woman! I'm going to call it: The Pussy Power Posse.* Emails were sent. Phone calls made. Women shared with other women. This was a grass roots effort. Eventually, small groups of women gathered in my tiny apartment's living room, month after month. Sharing their pains, desires, concerns, considerations, and more. Each gathering ended in smiles, gratitude, acceptance, and the feeling of being less alone. The circle grew and we moved to a community space. And soon, the community space expanded across the world. The PPP[1] (my affectionate name for the group) transitioned into the Rock Your Mojo®

---

1. My use of the word *Pussy* was ahead of its time. As much as I wanted to keep it, I took my business coaches advice, rebranded, and built all the Rock Your Mojo programs and live events. The commitment being to women getting what's possible with this work. And sometimes, that requires a more traditional, user-friendly doorway.

brand. Thousands of women have engaged in the virtual programs and live events over the years since then.

Hello, body. Are we ok?

Barbies and Ken dolls became my refuge. I loved making them do *grown up* things. Sweetly pressing their toy bodies together. Mushing plastic faces and making sweet kissy noises between them. I orchestrated the scenarios in my closet to escape the chaos of the domestically violent home that was my new normal with Mom's second husband. Maybe it was my way of creating scenes where a man wanted to be lovely to a woman. Where he fawned over her. Gave her genuine love, affection, and sexy time. These prepubescent passages became my signature trick during sleepovers. Under the fold out couches, in the tents made of sheets and blankets, or in empty bathtubs. I wanted to talk about this with all my girlfriends. I saw bawdy scenarios on late night TV watching The Benny Hill Show. They made me understand it could be fun and playful to enjoy someone else's body. I decided my friends needed to know about the wonders of that thing adults do. The thing I used to do with the boy across the street. The thing that gripped my brain and was one of the few things that made me happy.

Cut to five years later. Summer Camp in Fryeburg, Maine. I got breasts before most other girls. And they were big—fast. My menstrual cycle came early too. I was the first of the bunch[2]. The

---

2. The first time I got my period was on Christmas break in St. Croix. It was embarrassing, traumatic, and frustrating. I bled through my favorite pale pink cotton jeans at dinner, Mom's second husband continuously pounded on the bathroom door as she tried to teach me how to use a tampon, and I couldn't wear a bathing suit for a few days.

rafters of Cabin 8 became the platform for early sex ed and I was the teacher, at thirteen. How to use a tampon, what it's like to wear a bra, and kissing boys were on the curriculum. Where I got the Mojo and sheer Moxie to *teach* those things at that ripe age has no answer except—Soul Calling: the thing you are uniquely suited and destined for in this lifetime. As in, my mission this time around is to experience difficult things related to my body, sexuality, and *woman-ness*. Then, go through the process to heal them and share the wisdom with others. I believe this is why I was raped the first time I had sex.

I wanted to have sex. I even tried with a boy from school the month before the fateful night. Alas, he was (and probably still is) extra well-endowed and my virgin pussy was not having any of it. The man who did take my virginity was a local from town in his early twenties. I was a freshman. He broke into my room at boarding school and refused my incessant no's. I was petrified to get kicked out, that would mean going back to the abusive household I cleverly escaped with boarding school. The man had his way with me. I silently cried. Shame burrowed into my bones. I told no one. Until I made a short film about it six years later as a sophomore at NYU Film School. That broke my silence. That gave me access to my body. That cracked the shame and let the light back in.

Cut to seven years later. I'm married. At twenty-seven. To a nice man. A good man. A place to land kind of man. He just wasn't the turn-me-on-and-light-my-loins kind of man. Our two-year friendship morphed into our love affair in Paris (so on the nose, I know)! He was working on a film over there and I, recently departed from my fancy job in Hollywood to start a metaphysical business, was having an existential crisis. His spare bedroom in Paris seemed like a solid spot to breathe and dream into the next phase. Visioning what my new business would look like, how I would reach as many clients as possible, and the potential impact the business could have when all the parts came together were front and center when I thought of my respite in Paris. I never imagined the next phase would include him. The first six months were dreamy—the honeymoon phase can have that effect. Add in that we were bicoastal and flitting back and forth between LA and NYC made it all the more heady. Think big screen romance including the one time he shouted, *Hey! Deborah! I love YOU!* as he boarded the plane and all the passengers in the waiting area ended up applauding. It was pretty epic in the beginning. He proposed seven months in and at ten months, we were living in LA as husband and wife. We were a good team and great friends. But little by little, year after year, something went awry. He turned me off. My childhood trauma surfaced and we weren't equipped to right our sinking ship. My superficial need to drive the train, my masculine drive, became annoying—to me. I wanted a *man*. A dude. A partner who was the masculine drive. What I quickly learned in January of 2003, at a retreat that changed everything, was that as long as *I* was holding down the fort on the masculine drive side of the street, I made it virtually impossible for a partner to surpass my masculine essence. And at that stage of my life, I desperately wanted to embrace *the feminine*. We were divorced by the end of 2003 and I made new vows to and with myself.

Deborah, I vow to learn, embrace, embody, and own your juicy, alive, sensual, sexual, spiritual, and wholistic feminine power. I vow to do whatever it takes in whichever way is for the highest good of All.

The next five years altered everything and became the basis for the memoir pieces in this book. I studied with copious amounts of teachers, mentors, gurus, and books! I was fervently dedicated to and invested in my growth *as a woman.* Those years also gave me a variety of opportunities with a diverse assortment of lovers. Each time and with each one, I looked for the lesson. The growth. Where did I still trip up? Where did I want to shrink into the old, known parts? And more importantly, which were the keys that set me free from my shackles? I was determined to not only embrace the wild, juicy, feminine aspects. The critical link was to have them all connected to and in service of my Spirit. Because deep in my bones, down to the core of my being, *I knew* that everything was energy and that everything was connected. The idea that our Spirit wasn't, dare I say, the same as our Sex was not something I could ever claim as Truth. My intention throughout these pages is to help you find *your Truth.* The Truth of the connection to and expression of your sex and spirit.

Everything is Energy

My college boyfriend blasted open the metaphysical door for me. By turning me on to Khalil Gibran's *The Prophet,* giving me a necklace with my first gemstone, a round quartz crystal sphere suspended in a silver winged dragon that hung from a black leather cord, and helping me look beyond the surface layer of life, he blurred the lines between sex and spirit. The metaphysical books helped open my mind and soul. The gemstones taught me how to harness energy for healing, manifestation, and more. And endless conversations about spirituality and consciousness offered me the possibility of crafting a life by choice.

I remember one particular night when we made love and suddenly, I couldn't breathe. He was loving me with every fiber of his existence, pressing it into me through our sex, and everything around us became fuzzy. He effortlessly tuned me into *our breath*. He continued to love into me. I wept and felt, what could only be called *The Spirit*, move through our bodies. Nothing like this ever happened to me before. There had been a moment when I was having sex with my boyfriend senior year in high school where I felt like my body was dissolving. It had felt otherworldly and a bit crazy to me at the time. I had had a similar feeling under the gospel tent at the New Orleans Jazz Fest multiple times and in Al Green's church during Sunday service. That night with my college boyfriend, it was undeniable. There was something beyond the physical occurring. His steady, slow thrusts into me combined with his capacity to hold the space for what was emerging between us was nothing short of magically cosmic. It was as if all of our individual energy merged into each other, and then that collective energy expanded into *all* the energy in the world.

Energy. It makes up every single thing in the universe. I am no physicist, though I have read quite a bit about it, and I adore that science has confirmed what many metaphysical traditions and practices have touted for thousands of years. Everything is energy. What excites me the most about this is we are never actually stuck. Energy is constantly moving. It can shift in rate and frequency. But, it never stops. The good news about that is we can transform anything we desire. Including your relationship to yourself, your sexuality, and spirit.

There are many names for this energy of the universe. In Japan, they call it *ki*. In China, they call it *chi*. In India, they call it *prana*. In Europe, they call it life force. The Latin word, anima, is used to describe this "animating principle" in all life. As is the word *ruh* in Sufi literature. I call it Mojo. Your special sauce; your *sexual energy*.

Let's be clear—your sexual energy is not the same thing as sex[3]. This may be one of the most critical distinctions one can make in life. The freedom that comes from this understanding creates immeasurable possibility. Every single client of mine over the past twenty-five years shared that when they made this critical distinction, they no longer felt debilitating shame about their sexuality. Women also said that knowing their sexual energy is natural, and not the same as sex, gave them more freedom to tap into it daily. They felt that it gave them more energy and enthusiasm for life overall. And that it also translated into better relationships with their loved ones, co-workers, and friends.

Your sexual energy *is* the same energy that makes the moon move the tides. The same as the sun's rays feeding the plants. The same as the acorn's essence making an oak. Sex energy is the animating, always present force that moves life forward. And it is *in you*. The absolute mysterious perfection of that energy brought a sperm and an egg together, and now that's you. You are the incarnation of life force, aka sexual energy.

Napoleon Hill's 1937 best-selling personal development book, *Think and Grow Rich*, dedicates an entire chapter to the use of sexual energy. In it he says, "Those who lack sex energy will never be enthusiastic, nor inspire others with enthusiasm."[4] I was so excited reading those words for the first time that I nearly fell off my chair. It confirmed what I felt inside—we *must* have a relationship with this vital force and use it consciously. Additionally, the distinguished philosopher and spiritual

---

3. I created a four-part series on The Real Undressed podcast about this topic. You can listen to Part 1 here: https://therealundressed.com/245

4. Hill, Napoleon. *Think and Grow Rich*. The Random House Publishing Group, 2019. (pg. 188).

teacher, Omraam Mikhaël Aïvanhov says the following about it, "The sexual force is essential for life and is the one thing which can make you love life. Therefore, you must never suppress this force.[5]"

Eros and the Erotic

Eros is much more than the cherubic winged figure we see depicted in art. Eros is even more than what we refer to as the Greek god. Eros, like chi, ki, prana, and sexual energy, is life force. It is the creative sexual energy pulsing through life. It offers you the experience of wholeness. Of being connected to everything. Because, again, everything is energy and when you are living from this knowing, you are honoring your *erotic nature*.

The psychotherapist Esther Perel speaks about the erotic beautifully on an episode of the On Being podcast. She says, "It is about how people connect to this quality of aliveness, of vibrancy, of vitality, of renewal. And that is way beyond the description of sexuality. And it is mystical. It is actually a spiritual, mystical experience of life. It is a transcendent experience of life."[6]

When you claim your erotic nature, you become erotically alive, vibrant, and vital. And that is when your life turns technicolor. It is when pleasure becomes the norm and when you experience

---

5. Aïvanhov, Omraam Mikhaël. *Sexual Force or The Winged Dragon*. Editions Prosveta, 5th Ed. 1997. (pg. 35).

6. Tippett, Krista (Host), "Esther Perel – The Erotic Is an Antidote to Death" On Being, 11 July, 2019. https://onbeing.org/programs/esther-perel-the-erotic-is-an-antidote-to-death/.

the full body *yes* to life. Your erotic nature is yours for the having. It is already in you.

Power Centers

Your erotic nature, this inherent sexual energy that pulses in you, is channeled through and supported by seven main power centers of the body. Think of these like your local power company's transformers. They move the energy and facilitate its smooth distribution throughout the region. Your body's seven power centers do this in a similar way. They line up from the base of your spine up to your crown on a central channel. They all go from the front of your body to the back. Each center has a particular quality, essence, and general *flavor*. When you connect to, open, engage, and activate each center, your life force can easily animate your entire being. This is why it's beneficial to learn about these centers and begin to form a conscious relationship with them. Like many things I find the most valuable in life, your power centers are not a *one and done* type of engagement. They need patience, maintenance, practice, connection, and honoring. Your erotic nature wants to bloom open all seven centers. What can and does shut them down is trauma—mental, emotional, or physical. This is why it's critical to understand and cultivate your power centers. Because everyone, and yes, I'm going to say *everyone*, has gone through some kind of trauma. It's part of the human experience.

The power centers open and close. They are living, breathing aspects of you. When you attune to them it becomes easier to decipher which one is wilted, and therefore needs a bit of nourishment.

Rest assured, your power centers will be shut down at some point. They might be right now. And that's ok. It happens to all of us. The good news is they are energy—and remember, energy is constantly in motion. When one, some, or all of your power centers are closed for business, it is deliciously simple to reengage them. Let's be clear. Simple is not always *easy*. It takes a bit of effort, but every inch worthwhile.

Personal power, magnetism, and pleasure are yours for the having when you play with and open your power centers. It is then you are letting your life force bloom throughout your being. Like Omramm Mikaël Aïvanhov says, "You must never block your energies, but prepare channels so that they can flow and irrigate your land, just as the ancient Egyptians dug canals so that the Nile could irrigate their country."[7]

This book is a journey through the channels—called your power centers.

Your Invitation (*i.e., How to use this book*)

UNDRESSED: An Invitation to Claim Your Erotic Nature is divided into seven sections. Each one is based on one of the seven power centers. The sections open with a brief overview of the center. You are then offered an erotic tale. An amuse bouche. A slice of my life in which I experienced the essence of that particular center with and through a lover. Then, it's Your Turn. This is when you get to take the center for a spin utilizing sexual and spiritual practices.

---

7. Aïvanhov, Omraam Mikhaël. Sexual Force or The Winged Dragon. Editions Prosveta, 5th Ed. 1997. (pg. 50).

The stories all took place between 2004 and 2008. They are not shared in chronological order. Nor is that important. Each story is meant to stand alone as a representation of the awakening I experienced with that particular power center. Similarly, each story uses *he* and *I*. It could have easily been *she* and *I*. Gender is not the point. Awakening and embracing one's erotic nature can happen with anyone of any gender.

I am grateful to each of my lovers, but their names are not important. I did my best to share their essence while retaining their privacy. And truly, the intention with the stories is for you to fall into them and feel like this can happen to you too. Or to remember a situation when it has happened for you. Ultimately, the stories are meant to turn you on and ignite your erotic nature.

The Your Turn section offers you potent practices to awaken each center, sexually and spiritually. All the practices are ones I personally use to this day. And if you, like me, experienced any form of abuse, please go slow. Your awakening can activate old feelings. Trust yourself, and only stretch as far as comfortable. If needed, get support from a trauma informed counselor[8].

You may read the book from front to back. You may jump around. Either way, my strong recommendation is that you spend time with each section and its practices. One center per week is a good way to go. No matter what, be gentle, kind, and loving with yourself on this journey.

Overall, give yourself a chance to try this path. To claim your erotic nature. The only way to know if it's worthwhile is to take the first step. Take the bits that work for you and leave the rest.

---

8. You'll find some options in the resource section at the end of the book.

My desire is that you find more of yourself in these words, wrap yourself up in them, and let them become your superheroine cape. Here's to you! Let's do this. Let's get undressed.

GROUND

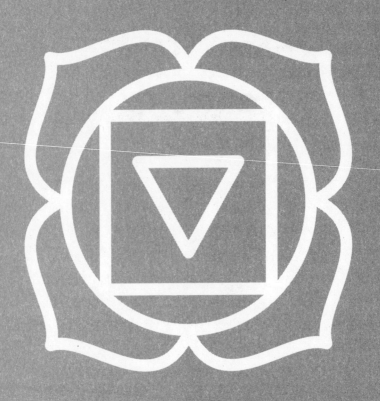

Power Center No. 1

ROOT

Color: **RED**

Sense: **SMELL**

Element: **EARTH**

Physical Location: **PERINEUM**

{the area between the anus and the vulva}

Objective

The Root Center connects you to the physical world. It is about your basic needs—food, water, and shelter. This center gives you basic instinct and survival skills. Its aim is to keep you in one piece, grounded, and alive. It is the foundation that allows you to go confidently forward and construct life. This center is the one most intimately connected with life force as it is the base for all the higher centers.

Harmony

Your Root Center is in harmony when you feel safe and secure, with yourself and life. Your erotic nature flows easily here. There will be an affinity with nature, Mother Earth, and all living things. You have an innate sense of trust in life with a healthy Root Center. It is easy to achieve your desires and there is comfort in the natural cycle of birth, death, and regeneration.

Disharmony

When your main focus is on making money, acquiring material possessions, or obsessing over your security, your Root Center is malfunctioning. If you are only thinking of yourself without considering others and excessively using sensual indulgences (such as sex, food, alcohol, or drugs), it's time to balance your Root Center. Additionally, when rage, anger, violence, or greed are your dominant expression it is a tell-tale sign that you are feeling insecure and operating from survival. Feeling sluggish, depressed, or unusually rigid are also signs of an off-kilter Root Center.

ARE YOU EXPERIENCED?

I can't trust a man who doesn't know how to fuck me. And I don't mean fucking as a technique. I mean fucking as a way to possess power. To exert power. To dominate. To physically and dynamically take control of another. The bare essence of raw sex stripped to its core.

I've had a lot of men over the years of all shapes and sizes. Some were sweet, gruff, talented, awkward, and everything in-between. Through all of them I continue to walk around with a yearning, a craving. The deep red desire that burns at the very root of me. I want to be claimed. I want to have the raw-blood-dripping-from-the-kill claiming that only a man can give me. There have been moments. Glimpses. Near connections where I'd dropped through the portal and was graced with the essence of being claimed. Yet, no one could sustain the stronghold. Until I met him.

It's 9:15 p.m. on a Tuesday night. I'm sitting at the local club drinking a glass of red wine. It's earthy and I like it. Half a glass is all it takes for me to loosen my bootstraps. The musician on stage looks like a friend from high school but sings like Chet Baker. Certain notes strike chords in my pussy, dusting it off from slumber.

Eyelids at half-mast, my body sways left and right bopping ever so slightly up and down to the music. The dimly lit room, about the size of four average living rooms put together, smells vaguely of French fries. People mill about, drinking, and chatting, which adds another layer of texture to the music.

I wasn't completely content. I felt antsy. Earlier tonight, I wanted something, like an epic adventure and at the same time, nothing, where sitting in silence could be ok. This bipolar state of being pulled me to wander out in the night. I threw on some shoes and a light shawl. Stepping out my front door into the balmy night, the moonlight slashed across my face as if to dissect me right there and then. She reminded me we are always in flux. Just like her. We grow full, we wane, we can feel utterly dark, and we rise to full-ness again. Over and over. Tonight, under her glare, it felt as though I was being ripped into a thousand pieces only to be tossed to the ground and become part of the Earth once again.

One by one, my sluggish legs carried me across the front path, down the slight incline of the hill and on through the little park that always makes me feel like I'm in Europe... or at least some-place foreign. The dew from the grass released thick musk from the dirt below. I thought about how I crave a man's scent. How I actually like to stick my nose into a man's armpit when we lie in bed. How much that turns me on—good body odor and phero-mones. When they're a match, there's nothing like it.

In the club, I smell him before I see him. Not literally his scent, but his presence is so deep that when I inhale, I know something shifts in the room. The lioness in me scans the terrain, observing move-ment while silently stalking new meat. Standing slightly over six feet at the back of the room, he's covered in a leather jacket and jeans. The red lights of the club reflect off his clean shaved head. His eyes remain clouded in mystery. He too seems to be scanning the room—a lion to my lioness. I don't feel an instant connection, but I know just by looking at him I'd like to get him in bed. He has presence. His body language says he knows he can have anything. All he has to do is take it.

I turn my attention back to the stage, swirl my finger around in the last taste of wine and suck it dry.

"You ready for another?"

He's standing right next to me with piercing blue eyes, sly smile.

"That'd be nice, but would you like to fuck?" I don't say it out loud, but I want too.

"Sure," slips through my lips. He motions to the cocktail waitress, raises my empty wine glass, and holds up two fingers of his other hand. Confidently, he positions himself on the bar stool next to me at the high-top table. Conversation is quick, with clipped sentences that seem like grunts.

"Where you from?" he asks.

"Big Apple. You?"

"Queens. Moved up the block a week ago."

"Mm."

"You live around here?"

"Yeah. You ride?" I motion to his leather motorcycle jacket.

"Yeah. Rode her across the country."

I silently nod, eyes brightening and lips twist into a wanton smirk.

"You wanna go for ride?"

"Yeah."

Do I ever. Motorcycles are a passion of mine. The thrill of all that vibrating metal between my thighs. The roar of the engine.

The elements streaking across my naked face. Wrapping myself up against the man controlling the bike. Yeah. I like to ride.

He walks me back to his apartment. It's simple with the basics. A bed, table, chair, bookshelf, lamp, TV, boxes of books, and personal items yet unpacked plus curtains that are on the floor in the corner, waiting to be put up over the windows. He opens the closet and hands me a helmet that fits, a jacket that's too big, and clear goggles—it's nighttime after all. We walk to the back of the building where his motorcycle resides. She's a beauty. A cruiser. 1600 cc of pure black lacquer and shiny chrome. High handlebars, whitewall tires, small sissy bar (that I like to refer to as the bitch bar) and a softtail. She still has a New York plate. As he gears himself up (helmet, gloves, etc.) he gives me his riding rules. Blunt. To the point. He tells me who's boss.

"No sudden moves... Don't hold onto my shoulders, waist and chest are ok... Keep your feet on the pegs... If we go down, you stay with me... I always get on the bike first and you always get off first..."

Yes baby. A man who knows—get a woman off first. As I listen to him, I realize my panties are damp. What is it about a man telling me what to do that's such a turn on? Is it that I'm forced to give up control? That it instantly triggers my vulnerability? My feminine core? I'm not one to normally get bossed around, but having this man run me through his rules of the road revs my engine. He completely claims his space and is taking me on his ride.

A little afraid and a lot hot, I ease myself towards him after mounting the bike. I place my hand on his chest and lean in close to him. My breasts firmly press up against his back. He reaches around with his gloved hand and grabs my ass pulling it closer to him. I have no choice but to slide forward in the seat. My hot box crashes into his lower back.

"Now we're ready to roll," he says.

We ride up the coast highway with the moon as our guide. The ocean permeates the air and the black asphalt below whips by, making it seem as if we're floating above the Earth. His body and the sheer magnitude of the bike below me are the only things keeping me grounded. That and the pockets of icy air slapping my face every few miles. My chin rests on his shoulder and I feel safe. I find my hand slowly rotating in a circle on his chest. His body soothes me and just as I think that he takes my hand and moves it to his inner thigh. I'm not quite sure what he wants me to do. Sensing my hesitation, he takes my hand and moves it up towards his crotch. He places it over his cock, thick and engorged, and squeezes my fingers around its girth.

He half turns back to me, "I can feel your heat on my back. You need to feel mine."

I want him to pull the bike off the road, throw me over it, and put out the fire blazing in my pussy. But he doesn't. He keeps riding in total control. Confident. Silently asserting his power.

It seems to be momentary alchemy that makes me feel connected to someone. There's an instant flash that happens. Like the moment I saw him earlier. It's not an everyday thing. It's not even a weekly or monthly thing. It's like magic, only real. I talk about this with friends and there's the constant discussion about whether this kind of fusion can be sustained for any length of earthly time. Most of us agree that it's vertical moments. The ones that penetrate deep to the core and sizzle an existing foundation. They blast open a new plane of living and basically leave you wondering where the hell they came from in the first place. You're never forewarned. There's no top of the hour prediction report offering insight of when and where these moments will occur. If there was, I surely would have tuned into it earlier that night. Moments like these are life's little intruders. They demand attention and leave you wanting more long after they are gone.

I don't know this man my legs are straddling, but I *know* him. I know his energy. I know he is what I'd been craving. The truth of that splatters bilious fear throughout my entire body. When presented with this desire I find myself recoiling like water in a hot frying pan. When, in fact, all I need is to unfurl. Give myself permission to be wide open for claiming.

He pulls off the road near an expanse of the ocean where it meets looming boulders. The salty water crashes onto the rock spewing spray into the cobalt night. I begin to feel shaky as if I'm in a state of hyperawareness. My breath booms in my chest, things around me appear extra crisp in my eyes and I can taste emotion.

When I was a child, I enjoyed lying in the sun at the beach. The rays penetrating my skin gave me comfort that I didn't feel from family. Enveloped in the elements, I felt safe. Taken. Claimed. The sun pinned me to the Earth, telling me I had to stay put or else. I thought it had magical powers because a pulsing always grew in my young loins. Wavelengths of unfamiliar energy moved into my body and I thought it strange at the time. Inevitably, after returning home and waiting for the still of night when I was sure everyone else was asleep, the natural activity was to mount my bed pillow, hug it tight to me, sway back and forth, up and down, wrapping my hands under the pillow to press the pillow harder, with more firm strength up into me until I felt "the ocean" flood my body. This left awed air in the room as if two animals mated. Primal yet stunning.

He puts the bike in neutral and turns off the ignition. A commanding look from him and I'm off the bike... right, I get off first. His long strong leg swings over the metal beast situating him upright. A subtle nod of his head and we're off to the lifeguard station fifty or so feet away. Once there, he gallantly holds out his hand indicating I should climb the small ladder to the platform. His hand scoops my ass and up I go. The ocean sounds a drum chant, rhythmic and haunting. Red-hot blood fills my veins—comforting and maddening. Feeling as though I'll melt over the railing loosely holding me up, his road warrior arms slip through mine, around the front of my waist and pull my back to fuse his front. His hand travels south, grasping my clothed pussy. I melt back into his chest, becoming liquid. My shoulders peel further away from my neck. He holds me up from my sex. I believe that the power of his hand has killed thousands of lovers before me. They fell to dirt as I am in this moment. This man holding my place of life and death knows the code. He has platinum access. The ocean roars, stars violently flicker, and suddenly I am lightning fast facing this man who now controls me top and bottom. His cobra tongue whips through my lips and presses into mine. *Whip, whoosh*. Deep, then retreats pressing and directing mine again. He releases my sex to grab a fistful of my hair from the root. I stare into his eyes wordlessly asking if is he the one. Fierce confidence shoots from his baby blues into my green eyes saying, "Don't question that. We're good. Here, now". He knows I know better. Brazenly kicking my foot wide, he places his feet between mine as if to fuck me through our clothes missionary style while standing. Breathless, we stare into each other until he releases our momentary trance. Without hesitation, he walks away from me and descends the ladder saying, "C'mon kitten. Time to hit the road." Wait? Did he just call me kitten? Oh yes, indeed he did. And I like it!

The ride back into town is a blur. I know the earth is below, sky above, and this man is in front of me. But who is he? And who have I suddenly become with him?

"I'm not ready for the night to end," the rogue words escape my mouth and charge his ear.

"Then it won't," he says, more of a command than a statement.

He has me guide us back to my place. When I start to point into the night air for which way to turn, he pulls my hand to his thigh.

"No pointing for directions. Tap me on the right thigh for a right turn and on the left for a left turn."

I tap his left thigh indicating the direction to take and then let my hand rest on him. Every morsel of me is enflamed. Hot. Bothered. Ready to ravage his meat, but I'm fighting something deep inside. I'm the one who truly wants to be ravaged. I want to be claimed. I already feel the deep penetrating force of this man despite the fact that he has yet to physically be inside me. The giant sense of him bleeds through each moment, making me realize the magnitude of confidence he has without condescension.

With a tap on his right thigh, we turn onto my street. "Half a block up on the right. Those red iron gates. That's me," I purr into his ear.

We take off our boots and gear at the front door. No words. No touching. No hesitations. I walk through the living room to the stereo and turn on my favorite nighttime radio program—Nocturna. World beats, hip-hop, and funk flood the already groovy atmosphere. He stands for a moment intently watching me. "Breathe. Pace. Create the space," I silently tell myself. I take the lighter from its designated spot, pop a few tea light candles in their holders, light them, and some incense. A veritable love den. That's what my home is like. Filled with textures—velvet, silk, sheepskins, suede, and leather; colors—soothing and stimulating in all the right places; and of course smells—incense, fresh market flowers, candles. Gliding into the kitchen, I pull a bottle of red wine from the shelf and the opener from the middle drawer. Before I can take a breath, he's behind me. Those stunningly sculpted arms surround me taking the bottle and opener from my hands. Pressing with a firm gentleness from his groin, he moves me forward until I'm up against the counter. Without a word, he holds me pinned while he extracts the cork from its hole. His long fingers are surprisingly elegant. The nailbeds slightly rounded. Clean. Clipped. I imagine them pinching my nipples. I imagine them in my mouth getting wet from my saliva and then again, pinching my nipples. My breath becomes shallow. He must feel this because, like the giveaway letter from Vanna White's electric word display, he turns me around completing the phrase.

"Glasses are in this cabinet," he says reaching behind me opening the cabinet door as though he has X-ray vision.

"Uh, yeah..." spills out of my dazed mouth.

He pours us each a glass and leads me back into the living room. A particularly soul shaking beat plays on the radio. My booty wants to groove. Hips shyly sway from side to side, trying to fight it at first. A twisted grin forms on his face. "Go ahead baby, dance for me." He takes the wine glass from my hand and puts his and mine on the side table and takes a seat on the couch. With shy confidence I stare into his eyes. A slight tilt of my head and furrowing of my brow only makes his grin bigger. He does that thing guys do when they show confident approval. That combo of knowing smirk and upward chin move. Clearly, I have no choice. I dance for him.

My hips move in a slow figure eight finding their groove. My shoulders make their move to match. My head begins to bop up and forward as arms and hands wind their way through the air. I can feel the intensity of his eyes on my body. It turns me on and lets me fall deeper into the dance, which quickly becomes somewhat of a moving trance. A ritual dance. I find myself standing on the sturdy wood coffee table in front of the couch offering myself to him. Body swaying, undulating as though I am the snake being called from the basket—called by him. Shoulders roll back, arching my chest to the heavens as my head tilts taking my upper body into a half backbend. Coming back upright, I see him on the couch. Only now he is bare-chested. His skin smooth, pale. Nipples, a perfect cherry pink, rest on his defined pectoral muscles. The most awing mark, that makes me pause from my dance, is his tattoo—a red dragon climbs his chest to his collarbones. It doesn't hurt that his biceps bulge and his abs are clearly visible. This man, this fabulous specimen of physical strength and beauty inspires me. His absolute masculine force drives my feminine juice into sweet abandon. I resume my dance—spiraling hips and chest all the way until I rest on my knees atop the coffee table. I lean forward rolling my shoulders back while pressing my face towards his. We are so close I can feel his breath on me. He never loses contact with my eyes. I tilt my head to the right. His eyes follow. Then to the left. His eyes follow. Sweeping my head from the left to the right, I pause in the middle of his chest. I have to touch him. I have to taste him. I want to be the dragon climbing his chest. I want to be on top of him. I want to surround him. I want to feel nothing but him penetrating every single part of me. He grabs a fistful of my hair from the nape of my neck and pulls my face to look at him.

"You want to play with the dragon, baby," again, it's a statement and not a question.

"Yeah," I unabashedly concur.

His other hand reaches for my throat. It excites me and scares me. He knows it. He knows I feel his control—and it turns me on. Our mouths connect and he kisses me deeply while holding me with force. I am not going anywhere without his command. I feel consumed in the best way.

When he stood next to me at the bar earlier, I couldn't stop feeling his energy drawing me in and him to me. As if that moment pulled us into a black and white smoke-filled time warp. It's 1930 and Marlene Dietrich is crooning, *Falling in love again / Never wanted to / What am I to do?... Like moths around a flame.* When we started talking I knew something was there and then later in the evening he said, "I know now that I went to that bar to meet you." Funny. The universe has a way of making sure certain people cross paths at just the right time. Life crossing. From one to the next. Have we known each other before? In another incarnation? Who knows for sure and I don't need to figure it out. What I know is that something in me is opening through this man. Something raw. And real. And gnarly in the best way.

Skin to skin and limbs wrapped all over one another, we are on my bed. Our breath falls in sync without trying. Spontaneous. Natural. Like the earth opening to sunrise. She never resists. She always gushes her dew feeling the heat. I feel him in me without having him *in me*. Suddenly, I'm scared. Not of him. Scared of the part of me that's coming home again. Like a glacier melting, powerful and loud, it shifts the shape of the land. It creates new terrain and that once standing glacier now flows through so many other spaces. It feeds and nourishes the spots that might otherwise have gone arid and stayed craggy. The water gives life. It's cleansing.

I find myself silently asking for the strength to root into my I AM presence. To walk through this with honesty, integrity, compassion (for myself), and to know the difference between what's opening my soul and what, if anything, shuts her down. I ask to stay in my feminine presence, especially because this is a man that sees me and not one iota of him is threatened.

And then *whack*! A spiritual spanking crosses my psyche, dropping me to the shit stain on my ego's floor. I can hear that damn heckler laughing his way out of the not-so-tightly closed door of my mind.

The heckler. The one-man itty bitty shitty committee living inside my head opens his foul mouth with a wicked laugh, "*Bwah-hahahaha! Don't even think this is something special. You know you're not enough,*" he growls with cigarette-tinted saliva dripping from his hideous mouth.

"*Not now. You can't be here now,*" I silently whisper.

"*Oh yeah. You know I'm the one that has your number. I drive this trip. And you m'dear, Are. Not. Enough.*" The words pierce every inch of me. My heckler stating the real fear: Am I enough?

"*Fucking perfect,*" I hiss to the slovenly heckler. "*I'm perfect. You almost got me. Not this time.*" The words come easily for a change.

Like a fiery red phoenix rising from the ashes, I understand *this* man, the one whose flesh and limbs are entwined all over me. His power gives me power to stand up to my heckler and explore what's available right here and now with him. This man who fills me with his mere presence is the instigator for the electric energy dancing up and down every ounce of me. He inspires my body into the kriya shakes. The kind that looks like someone with their finger in an electrical socket—a body wracked by rapid undulations and staccato movements dancing up and down every ounce of me. This man is here to show me my fear in service of dissolving it. He is the mirror for me to see what's possible when one roots into themselves. When you feel fear and boldly walk forward anyway and when you honor the grit *and* the glory.

Right now, bringing my presence and consciousness back to the room where I am safely pressed into the dragon chest and wrapped in his potent arms, what I know for sure is this man has the power. This man knows me by nature. This man, well this man is a man I can trust.

"We have to be careful you know," he says with sleep in his eyes. The sun barely peeks through the window indicting a new day and the rumpled comforter, twisted like a Cirque du Soleil performer around us reveals our night of being piled, plowed, and spooned together despite the fact that we did it all without actually *doing it.*

"How so?" I say brushing a handful of hair from eyes.

"We're going to sleep together. Actual sex," he states.

"Oh we are, are we?" I giggle tugging at the comforter for extra cover.

"Yeah. We're Aries. We really enjoy each other, physically and more. Don't pretend to think that when someone like us has their mind on something that it can be avoided. There's no stopping people like us from getting what we want," again, a statement and zero question in his tone.

"I see. And why do we need to be careful?" I reply wriggling my leg between his to get our bodies even closer.

"Because you and me, we're meant to be in each other's lives for a really long time. It might not be what you think, but it's going to be for a long time. So, let's not fuck it up."

His eyes are clear, firm, and filled with the promise of love.

I get it. Even if this whirlwind encounter doesn't turn out to be my fantasy of what might be possible with this man, that he may not be MY man; I get it. There's a mystery unfolding between us. Bigger than a romance, something essential with consequences that can elevate who we are for each other and for ourselves. In this moment, it's eminently clear that all there is to do is surrender to each other's power. And I'm grateful. I am forever shifted and newly rooted in I AM. I know I can be met. I know I can have a powerful man. I know I can be sacred and profane. I feel safe, sexy, and hot.

With as much playful cooing as I can muster, I look to find the space behind his eyes, the place where we *know* each other, and do that thing making my chin move upward and lips smirk knowingly and I say, "Well then Sir, let's not fuck it up."

YOUR TURN

Root Center

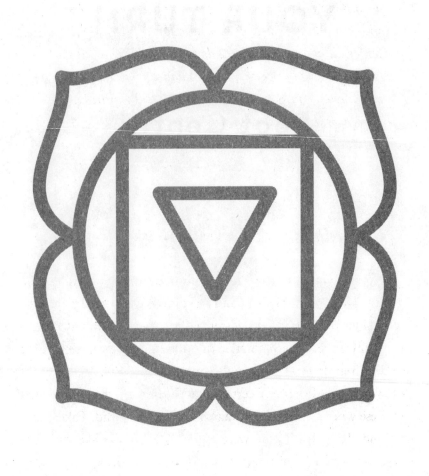

*The Root Center is the power center of raw primal urges,
animalistic nature, and uninhibited qualities. The Root
Center is the transition point between our animal life and
our human one. It's about our relationship to the Earth
and the material world. When functioning well, the Root
Center allows you to have a depth of purpose in all that
you do. On the contrary, an imbalanced Root Center is
only focused on survival and fulfillment. Primordial life
energy and the ability to trust play a main role in this
center. Stability, the power to achieve, and physical will
of being are all experienced here.*

To access its depth, we're going to play with the ass.

Now, if you're like me you might be squirming reading this.
Ugh. My ass. I mean it's dirty and all sorts of potential embarrass-
ment resides there. I feel you sister. Here's the deal though. In order to fully experience the magic of your Root, we must embrace
the taint (it ain't your ass, it ain't your pussy).

For instance, I'm pretty certain that in this very moment as you
read these words, you're clenching your butt. Go ahead. Take a moment and check it out. You were, right? Well, you're like most humans. We walk around, sit at our desks, get ready, go grocery
shopping, hang with gal pals, go to the movies—and we are unconsciously contracting our asses. And not just our glute muscles, our
sphincters get in on the party. Your level of stress can be measured by
how easily you can get a finger in your ass. Nearly impossible? You're
Defcon 10 on the stress meter and your Root Center is suffering.

You might be thinking, so effin' what?! What's a tight ass (and not the physically fit kind) got to do with me having a deeper connection to my power and pussy? Well m'dear. Every-fuckin'-thing is what. This power center is the gateway to you trusting in life and yourself. When you were a kid your ass and all its functions were super fun to explore. Then someone told you—NOPE! Danger zone. Dirty zone. One-way zone. And your body took that information and began many years of clamping your ass down into a tight ball of nerves. I refer to these energetic neurobiological clusters as *kinks*, not the fun sex kind, but the detrimental kinks that hold you back from being free and self-expressed. We all have them, and they are in the way of experiencing your full potential (in and out of the bedroom).

Like the proverbial, *the universe has your back* shiznit, a high vibing Root Center gives you confidence in yourself and the world at large. The opposite of this is running around in fear, worry, and doubt—and that shit bleeds into our personal, romantic, and yeah, even business relationships. It has you on edge wondering who or what is going to take advantage of you. It's not a fun place to hang energetically, mentally, spiritually, or sexually.

Let's take this to a level of energy. In the quantum fields, it is a fact that everything is energy. That includes YOU... and your ass. When your ass's energy is all jacked up in knots, you will experience more nervousness, aggravation, and frustration. This is because the Root Center is located in this physical area. When it's energetically kinked up (meaning, not free flowing) you have the shadow side of the center.

Opening up to your ass and all that's available through this Root Center portal is where you access the light side of the center.

Confidence, raw sexual expression, and more, are your natural state when you're located in this space.

Let's get you cozy-connected to this portal in order to claim you're the shit (pun intentional). Not in an ego-based way, but in the way where you are sourced from the depths of your being, rooted in the potency of the universe.

Spirit Tools:

The following items can balance and invigorate the Root Center. Use them prior to your practice to set the tone. You increase your spiritual sexual connection by combining these spirit tools with the sex ones listed below.

◌ Anointing with Essential Oils

This is the practice of smearing or rubbing your body with a substance to bless and consecrate your body as a sacred, energetic space. It connects the physical with the spiritual. It's most typically done with essential oils.

> REMEMBER: Use a carrier oil if you have sensitive skin.
> Almond, coconut, jojoba, and olive oils are all good choices.
> You use a few drops of the essential oil with the carrier oil to
> make it easier on your skin and still reap the benefits.

Root Center: dot the base of your spine (aka the top of the crack of your ass)

Oils to use*:
- Patchouli (grounds, stabilizes)
- Vetiver (calming, rooting)
- Myrrh (increases awareness)
- Cedarwood (calming, grounding)

Elevating the Vibration with Crystals

Using crystals (forms of minerals from the earth) goes back as far as Cleopatra turning black eyeliner into a trend for the masses. Have the crystals in the room where you choose to practice, sitting, near or on your body.

Crystals to use*:
- Red Jasper (grounding, stability, strength)
- Red Garnet (rooting, energy enhancer)
- Black Onyx (releases negativity, enhances protection)
- Smoky Quartz (grounding, forward movement)
- Hematite (stability, embodiment)

Create the Mood with Music*

Music is energy created by sounds, each possessing a specific frequency. You know when a certain song gets you *in the mood*. Your body lights up. You feel a surge of sassiness. You might even feel your inner Bad Girl peek her stiletto out from behind your closeted psyche. If you choose to play music during your practice, make sure it *opens* you up. You'll know if it does when the pores on your body seem as though they are plumping up—like when your cheeks flush after someone says that particular sweet, naughty something in your ear.

Music to play:
* Anything that has real bass and drum always does the Root Center right. Music that focuses on the color red or fire in the lyrics is also a fun option. Most importantly, get the tunes that enhance *your* practice. It's all about you being IN your body experiencing power and pleasure.

Sex Tools*:

The following items are where it's at to get your Root Center alive and kickin' through ass play. I recommend practicing with them all, but not all at once. We don't want your sweet cheeks to go into shock. Each tool provides a specific nuanced sensation, thereby helping you reach a new threshold in your capacity for power and pleasure.

Lube

Don't even think about skipping this one. Ass play without lube is like being stuck in rush hour traffic. There's nowhere to go and feelings of homicide are normal. Let's keep it on the sexy, smooth side of the street. Lube, lube, and more lube ladies!

Remember, your body is a temple. Use healthy products free from glycerin, parabens, and other toxins. And please!!! DO NOT use lubes with flavors or heat enhancing properties (unless you like the feeling of a fiery ass).

Butt plugs and dildos

Size matters. In this case, smaller is better to start. Make sure to get one that has a flared base. This helps hold it securely in place and eases the extraction process when you're done playing. Choose one in a material that pleases you. There's a wide variety out there. I recommend ones you can clean easily like silicone, glass, or stainless.

Vibrators

The sex toy industry has come a long way since I was a kid. That's great news for all of us! Today, you can find vibrators specifically designed for anal play. The common vibrator is made for the vaginal canal and has different sizes and shapes. Anal vibrators are usually shorter in length yet can still vary in girth. Start slow and see where you end up taking it.

Hand towel

I recommend having a small stash that is exclusively for sex play. You can get these at any discount home goods store. This way you have dedicated clean up material that are washable and won't have you stressing out that you got some bunk on the good family linens.

✧✦ Permission:

Give it to yourself.
It's underrated and makes a world of difference.
I am giving you permission right now.
You are worthy of owning your erotic nature.
Now claim it for yourself.
Say it aloud: *I AM worthy of owning my erotic nature.*

By saying these words you are free to experiment and play with yourself, relish in your sexuality and connect it to your spiritual self. You are giving yourself a gift by doing so and therefore, you are opening yourself as a gift to the world. When you flourish, everyone around you will as well.

SOLO PLAY:

MIND

Wherever you stand in your position on ass play, it's important to open your perspective (even if only a teeny-weeny bit) to the fact that anal play can be incredibly satisfying and transformative. The opening of your ass is filled with nerve endings available to incredible amounts of pleasure. And just a mere two knuckles of an index finger inside gives you access to a whole new world of sensation connected to your pussy. Honey, if you've never had your clitoral roots stimulated through your ass...you're in for a delicious surprise. (FYI—the nub of nerve endings most women know of as the clitoris is literally the tip of the iceberg. There's a whole world underneath that, including the clitoral bulb and roots extending approximately four inches down[9]).

You might need to get over the idea that the ass:

* is a forbidden zone
* is a one-way street
* is dirty, noisy, or disgusting

---

9. Here is a link to a terrific diagram showing the layers of the clitoris: https://www.anatomyofpleasure.org/over-the-skin-what-you-can-see

- is going to cause pain sexually
- or any other tale you've been told

Consider the fact that ass play can open you up (literally and figuratively) to a realm where confidence, personal power, and deep surrender exist.

BODY

Preparation makes for a pleasant experience. Therefore, especially if you are new to ass play, setting yourself up for success is key. That starts with a clean canvas. Get out those baby wipes or get busy with your bidet or hand shower. Give that sweet ass a nice rinse. It'll make you feel fresh and your pussy will be clapping because she's not interested in swapping bacterial microbes with your booty. For those of you who are really "anal" about your cleanliness, yes, pun intended, an extra step is to use an enema beforehand for that extra sparkling clean experience.

Next, make sure you've got uninterrupted time. At least thirty minutes is a good container to begin experimenting. Make sure you have all of the suggested tools you want to use nearby.

Claim this practice as sacred time with one, some, or all of these suggested intentions. Say them aloud with as much Mojo as you can muster.

- ✧ It is safe to explore my erotic nature
- ✧ Being erotically alive feels good
- ✧ It's good to be erotically alive
- ✧ I am open to exploring my sexuality
- ✧ I am open to the possibility of pleasure through my ass

✦ My ass is a source of erotic bliss
✦ When I open and relax my ass, I am opening to experiencing power and pleasure
✦ I love being sexually and erotically vibrant
✦ Every part of my body is sacred and sexy, including my ass

Get into a comfortable position. This varies so make sure it works with your particular body. You could be on your back with knees bent pointing to the ceiling. You could be on your side or on your belly. Getting on all fours is also a great position for ass play. Find the position that enhances the moment, not one that's going to distract you.

Start with your fingers (a bit of lube on them is helpful. Grab a small scoop or a generous squirt of your preferred kind). Imagine you're Jacques Cousteau searching for treasure in foreign waters. Find the opening of your ass. Place one or a few fingers on it.

Breathe. Breathe again. And once more. Consciously connect to this space on your body that you are 99 % of the time unconscious towards. Once you've made this energetic *Hello*, start to press, flick, strum, knead or any other gesture your finger(s) feel inspired to make on the opening of your ass. What about the surrounding skin? Don't forget about that. Does she enjoy a light stroke? A little pinch? What about dancing back and forth between the flesh just outside the opening of your ass and the opening itself? When you feel a bit turned on, take a finger and insert it into your sweet ass. Start slow. One or two knuckles should do it. Breathe. Get used to the sensation of something entering INTO your ass. Most likely, your default reaction rears her head to clench down and tighten (it's normal and very fight or flight mode). Instead, choose to open. Expand. Trust.

Once you let your fingers do the ass talking dance, trust in yourself increases and you might find that you start doing other things that previously felt off limits (learning to ride a motorcycle anyone?!). Each and every time you do the unthinkable, your courage grows, and fear shrinks. You flex your Mojo muscles, release shame, and silently shout a resounding YES to life.

At this point, you can move your finger in and out, rotate it slowly in a circle, pulse it down or up or sideways. The whole point is to discover what brings you a bit more alive and provides the next level of opening in your Root Center.

When you feel satisfied with finger play, you're ready to incorporate a vibrator and/or butt plug.

A vibrator can be used just like your finger, however make note to keep a firm grip on it. You wouldn't want your ass to clench up and suck it in too far.

Butt plugs! Oooh baby, you're in for a treat! First thing to note, as mentioned previously, you need to use one that flares at the base of it. Just like when you started with your fingers, you absolutely want to have a good amount of lube available. Have some on the opening of your ass and on the plug.

Then, tease the opening of your ass a bit with the tip of the plug. Think of it like a bit of foreplay. When you feel ready (well, as ready as you'll be), gently begin to press the plug into your ass. Breathe. Deep breaths are extremely helpful here. With each exhale, let your ass relax and bloom open. The plug will *slip in* once you are relaxed. At that moment, the only thing to do is pause and connect to the sensation of it. Feel the weight. The pressure. The fullness. Consider how you feel. Awkward? Good? Turned on? Annoyed? Surprised? Notice what the sensation of a butt plug in your ass brings up. This gives you clues to where you've been clenched (or open). Once you're acclimated to the plug, you have a few options:

- Enjoy the sensation of the plug for a few moments in sync with deep breathing.
- Keep it in and do some slow hip circles. You can do these standing up or on your hands and knees. This lets you connect to the Root Center and generate life force energy together—a potent combo offering you that deeper level of confidence.
- Keep it in and go about your business. Literally. Go read/send some emails, wash the dishes, make the bed. Let the plug be the reminder to open, experience pleasure and be connected to your Root Center.

When you're complete with your plug, slide it out of you *on an exhale.*

Bonus tip: Place the plug in a hand towel you keep nearby. Don't worry if there's anything on the plug. You need to wash the plug regardless. Keep your plug (and all sex toys for that matter) clean. A natural soap and some water will do the trick or you can use one of the many toy cleansers available.

SPIRIT*:

Sit in a quiet space where you can be undisturbed for five to fifteen minutes.

Light a candle if that inspires or feels good to you. A red one symbolizes the Root Center. In addition to the candle, incorporate any of the additional spirit tools you are drawn to use for this meditation.

Gently close your eyes and begin by taking three deep belly breaths.

Let your low belly expand with your breath. Really stretch your belly out by how much breath you are receiving—like, let your low belly be deeply pregnant with breath. Once you are connected to your body, begin to imagine a low hum sound coming from a far-off place. It continues to increase in volume as it gets closer to you. When it is just in front of you, allow it to enter and rest in your Root Center. Notice the sensations. You might experience a tingling. You might feel a slight weighted vibration. Or you might feel nothing. Any or all of this is perfect.

Continue to breathe deeply.

The low hum stays in your Root Center as it expands directly down into the floor or ground below you. It drops deeper and deeper and deeper into the very core of the Earth. Imagine you are supported by the very essence of life. The same energy that allows the grass to grow and the flowers to bloom is cradling you through this invisible sound cord.

Take three deep belly breaths.

Now, consider all the thoughts, feelings, words or beliefs that keep you from experiencing pleasure and power. Allow them to travel into your Root Center. As soon as they reach the Root Center, the vibration of the low hum extinguishes them like candles on a birthday cake. They instantly lose power.

Take a deep breath.

Now, the low hum cord continues to vibrate as it's anchored in the core of the Earth. From here, the very center of the Earth, you begin to see a red ball of light. It may bounce, flicker, or simply be still. Allow that red glow of light to connect to the base of your low hum cord. It begins to grow. It expands upwards on the cord. It feels soothing and warm. It continues to climb up the cord all the way until it reaches your Root Center.

At the Root Center it pauses. It pulsates. And it eventually expands horizontally like a round, living disk of light. It is your new seat. Your throne. It is the regal Root Center here to support you in all ways.

When you feel complete, pull the hum cord up from the center of the Earth. Let it coil around the perineum, like a hose, on your red seat. Do this at whatever speed naturally occurs. Once the cord is coiled, take three deep breaths. Connect to the knowing and the sensation that your power is here. Right now. You have direct access to life force. You are supported here and now.

Gently flutter your eyes open.

Welcome back.

* *Visit www.undressedbook.com for your free downloadable resource lists and guided meditation*

SEED

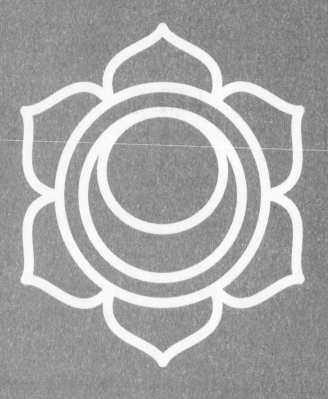

Power Center No. 2

LIFE FORCE

Color: **ORANGE**

Sense: **TASTE**

Element: **WATER**

Physical Location: **LOW BELLY**

{the entire space below the navel and above the pubic bone}

Objective

The Life Force Center is where all of creation lives. This is the space that manifests, brings forth, and generates new life. It is instinctual and associated with emotions. It desires to relinquish the ego and instead, merge with another. Interpersonal relating lives here, particularly, intimate union. It is part of the always evolving nature of the universe. It expresses itself as creative and deeply feeling.

Harmony

You experience ease and grace with your erotic nature. You feel the surge of life force moving through your body, soul, and mind. Intuition is the name of your game and it's spot on more often than not. You are continuously awed and moved by the perfection of life. Enthusiasm is your baseline. You easily flow with life and enjoy connecting with people. Sexuality and sensuality are your friends, free of shame or judgement.

Disharmony

There is no childlike wonder to your life. Sexual connections are either nonexistent or misused and unsatisfying. Emotions tend to be out of control with frequent outbursts. You are unable to maintain healthy boundaries and people tend to take advantage of you. There's no *zing* to your life and you feel mired in your problems. You are not comfortable in your body.

Do Me, Baby

The Metro North train lumbers along its route. Final destination—Manhattan's Grand Central Station. An eye on my suitcase in the little slot near the train doors, I decide it's time to relax and flip through a magazine. I'm coming from a conference in Boston and making my way to the city to see some consulting clients. Despite the cool November air outside, the train car is moist with life. Packed full with daily commuters and other passengers on their way to God-only-knows-where to do God-only-knows-what. I play a game with myself, where I try to imagine what each person does or where they're going. Maybe even where they came from. Who had a fight with their spouse/lover/family member/friend this morning? Who had sex? Who is sick? Who's coming from or going to visit someone who's sick? On and on it goes in my mind, dreaming up scenarios, simple and grandiose. All to pass the time and take my mind away from the malaise that doesn't want to let me go.

Existential crisis. That's been the theme in my world for the last few months. I'm due for a spat of it. It tends to come around when I feel misaligned in life. When I am not sure I know what I'm doing. Or why I'm doing it. The days and nights keep flowing and it all seems meaningless. The bottom line question consistently shows up as: what am I doing with my life? How can I best serve? Times like this tend to be the low points for me because, like most people, I have a desire to create. To bring forth beauty, light, power, pleasure, love, and inspiration. When my creativity plug is out of its socket, I seek out creative instigators. Thinkers. Feelers. Artists. Philosophers. That's why I'm going down the Anais Nin rabbit hole and listening to a few of her lectures from the early 1970s. She spoke about how people have always wanted to tap into awareness, reveal one's spiritual nature, and learn how to shine from their soul selves. Then, I happen upon Larry King Live where he spoke to a panel about the power of positive thought and their discussion about creating your own reality. I can feel the truth of that lodged in a dark corner of my body. I need help to bring it out.

Dada dun da dundun dun... my cellphone begins its perky Parliament Funkadelic ring tone. Searching for a ringing cell phone on a crowded train can be like bobbing for apples at a carnival. You never look cool and the damn thing always slips out of your hand at least a few times before you victoriously pull it up.

"Hello, this is me." I chirp, wrangling the phone to my face.

"Baaaaby. Is that you? Really you?"

His voice lands straight in my loins. It still has that seductive lilt.

"Oh wow. Hi. Yes. It's me. Is that really you?!"

Of course I know it's him. How could I not? He's forever embedded in the fabric of my life. The kind of way back you're happy to revisit.

"I just woke up and played my messages. And lemme tell you it was so good to hear your voice. Where are you? Are you in NY?"

I was 18 years old, two and a half years into a full sexual life—meaning I'd been getting laid for two years, when I first met him. I came home from boarding school for the weekend as I tended to do. I can't remember if I was set up on a date or if I'd met a man, and then we arranged the date. Either way, I found myself sitting at the bar of Banditos Mexican restaurant on Second Avenue and 10th Street in the East Village. I wasn't interested in my date who was quickly becoming liquid in his chair from one too many. I was interested in the bartender. He was electric. Beaming. Brilliant. Standing at a lean 6'1", his chocolate brown corkscrew curls cascaded past his shoulders onto the upper part of his chest, which stood at full attention. His chest poured smoothly to his slim waist creating that triangle shaped upper body—the kind that's perfectly done and not the overbearing one where you wonder how a man with that shape can actually move from one side to the next.

"More fruit juice?" he smiled from behind the bar.

"Sure."

I was in a phase of not drinking alcohol; hence, juice at a bar.

"Hey, what's with the guy?" He tilted his head in the direction of my date who just stumbled off to the bathroom.

"Dunno. Just met him."

"So you're single?"

"Ah, yeah. I guess so."

"Good. What are you doing later?"

"Later? Not sure yet."

"Well, why don't you come meet me here at the end of the night... I close at 4."

"4 a.m.?"

"Yup."

Growing up between a New England boarding school and New York City cultivated an interesting sense of sexual identity. At boarding school, you didn't want to blend in, yet you didn't want to be "too much" either. Being "too much" meant you were a slut. Easy. Your reputation came before you and no matter if it was true or not, the words would ultimately be your downfall. In New York City, you could be whoever you wanted to be. And it seemed that being bold, brazen and rooted in a budding sense of power was wildly admired. Come to think of it, these opposing sentiments perfectly echoed my understanding of sexuality fed to me from childhood. Demure behavior, good! Breezy sexual independence, good! Which one to be? And when?

"I'm on the train going to the city now."

"Wow. Baby. How's married life? How many kids do you have now...?"

"Whoa whoa... we really haven't talked in a while," I chuckle. "Babe, I've been divorced for 3 years now. And there are no kids."

We used to keep in sporadic touch for many years after we first connected for that 4 a.m. carnal adventure. Conversations on landline calls (it was the late 80s after all) morphed into our missives in emails in the early 90s and always the occasional in person connect when I would cruise through New York after moving to LA. Pending on our relationship status, the in person connects weren't always sexual. One time in late Spring, we sat in Washington Square Park eating deli food out of brown paper bags. One time we ate off each other's plates at the hippie health food joint in St. Mark's Place. Many times we had disjointed conversations as I sat at whatever bar he was tending. And one time we took a mini get away to Jamaica. I miraculously got two free airline passes when there was a complication with my luggage on a previous trip. My young, romantic self thought it very grown up to flit off somewhere with him. With quite a bit of planning that included him having to get his very first passport since this was his first international trip, we managed to pull it off. Every day on the island started with eating fresh papaya, mango, and pineapple. Playful romps in the sea and exploring the local sights took up most of the day. Evenings included fresh, exotically spiced foods and ended in delicately maneuvering our sunburns while having sex.

His life streamed forward with playing bass in the band that toured up and down the east coast, to his travels around the world inspired by our Jamaican get away, to his return to the States where he once again, recreated his reality to be exactly what he desired—a working musician and business owner. He was undeniably the one person I knew over the years that always oozed creativity and pure life force. Besides his obvious brawn, it was his energetic imprint that kept my keen interest and bringing me back into his orbit.

My entire body lit up talking to him. His words were fueled by utter focus and passion—two of his signature qualities. They spilled over the phone into my body, which instantly perked up and beamed sex energy into the already bright morning. I gushed pheromones and I could feel my pussy wanting to clap.

Fucking for fucking's sake intrigues me. It does not fulfill me. It's maintenance at best. The physical action is only rote. What I seek is something more. More from me and more from the one I choose to share my body with.

You see, that fateful night when I was 18 altered the way I experienced sex. Not just sex. But the way *I felt* about sex. My teenage brain had it all tipsy topsy since being raped three years prior. Rape being my first experience with penetrative sex. I was wanting to have sex—just not that way and not with that person. The experience left me numb, feeling like sex was obligatory and my body was something to be used.

I did go back to his place in the wee hours of that night we first met. He lived on MacDougal Street in the Village. It was a walkup. The loft space, divided up by bohemian curtains denoting each person's private sleep area, was fascinating to me. I'd never seen anything like it, but I could sense it was a place where people were up to things. Where life was intentionally made. Where desires came to fruition. With each breath, I wanted to inhale the essence of this lifestyle. The one that spoke so loudly of a vision pulling you rather than the textbook version of being pushed towards something prescribed.

That night was one exhilarating surprise after the next. He played bass for me. He took his time making the first move. He spied my inner turmoil about being with him sexually before I was conscious of it. He assured me I was safe—and without reason, I believed him. So much so, that I shared about being raped. It felt like the right thing to do. Maybe because I didn't want to seem like a prude after sitting at his bar only hours earlier. Maybe it was to erect a faux protective bubble and have an excuse to get out, just in case. His response was stunning. After denigrating the guy, he said, "Let me show you how it's supposed to be, ok? Let me give you pleasure. Let me change it up so you have a good experience of sex." I cried hearing his words. He brushed my tears away with his thumb. Then, he loved and sexed me up for hours and hours until the sun was high and we eventually fell into a deep sleep.

✧✧✧

"So you're single!!!" he cheers. I think everyone on the train can hear his enthusiasm blasting through the phone.

"Yeeeaaaah... are you single?" I ask with hesitation.

"Oh yeah! When do I get to see you?"

With my loins burning bright orange, we make plans to meet up in a few hours for a bite to eat. I need to sit with him. Breathe him in. Ingest his lust for life. It's exactly the antidote for my moody life malaise. My body is beaming with pure longing for him and what he possesses—unfettered creative juice. That and unconstrained sexual magnetism. We undeniably had it when I was 18. But that was 17 years ago. Is it possible that we're still that hot for each other now?

After I settle in and freshen up at my best friend's place, which is my steadfast NYC home away from home, I go to Lanza's Italian Restaurant on 2nd Avenue in the East Village to meet him. He first suggested meeting at his apartment, which I felt oddly nervous about.

"Oh babe, I didn't mean to make you uncomfortable," he had said on the phone, echoes of his care and consideration from that first night wafted through my psyche.

"No, no. It's not that. I, I just want to sit with you for a bit. Look at you and breathe."

There's something about him in my memory that always feels kind of *dramatically* creative. He always wants to make the moment memorable and does the most he can for you to feel special in it. Like that one time when I was feeling down and he sent me a pep talk video. He told me to save it for whenever I needed the reminder.

And he's unwaveringly held his position in the top three (if not the number one spot). The top three comes from the age-old question, "Who's the best you've ever had in bed?" Without a flinch, a blink of my eye, or a pause in my response—his name always comes right out. I don't know if it's because our first time was when I was younger and therefore more impressionable. I don't feel like it's that. The very few times we've seen each other over the last 17 years I have always felt fireflies igniting each cell in my body whenever I stood next to him; whenever I thought of him too. Besides the sexual healing he opened in me all those years ago, his aura and sheer life force offer a potent transmission to anyone in his orbit. That is, if you're lucky enough to be awake and catch his vibe.

The last time we connected, he and I met for a friendly meal. I was married at the time. We at a cozy Middle Eastern café in the East Village where we talked and talked and stared into each other's eyes and he fed me with his fingers. Sex without sex. Steamed vegetables with tahini sauce. It didn't matter. A perfect orange carrot perched between his thumb and index finger coming towards my mouth. He could've fed me bloody steak (I gave up meat in 1991). I'd have eaten it. How can I be *this* electrified by *this* man and not my husband? The question streaked through my mind like a naked guy dashing onto the football field mid-play. Unavoidable and annoying. The questions continued to dash back and forth. How can I be having this meal, or *any* intimate interaction with *any* man that is not my husband? Was this morally questionable? Of course. Can I learn from it? Absolutely.

I sat there, across from that man, not just wild with yearning, but wild with life. Inspiration, excitement, and sheer enthusiasm raced through me like a thoroughbred. A raging river of ideas, thoughts, desires, projects, and female power surged my system. Why didn't I experience this in my marriage? That haunted me at the time. Somehow the struggle in my deepest core raged. I ached to be claimed—mind, body, and soul.

Five years have passed since I saw him. In the cab to the restaurant I wonder what he'll look like now. Did he age well (he's only five years my senior)? Did he do well in his life? Is he happy? Will I feel the same way about him now? I have the taxi drop me off one block before the restaurant. That way I can collect myself and find my footing.

The street is comfortably filled with eclectic people. New York City in the late Fall always excites me. Leaves scatter the concrete jungle—amber, carnelian, and dark cherry. The air sultry, is filled with foreplay. As if actors on cue, we approach the restaurant at the same time. I recognized him by his walk— deliberate, a mellow strut. Those long blue-jean-covered legs carry his leaner, but still stunning torso. He's wearing a black leather jacket. At the exact moment I register his face, he realizes it's me gliding towards him in a Marilyn Monroe cut cream belted swing jacket.

"Baaaaaby!"

Without breaking his stride, he scoops me into his arms. Oh my. His hands press into my lower back, mine wrap around his neck—now bare from his long locks that have been shorn into a thick piece-y Rockstar cut. I still have to stand on my tip toes, even in heels, while hugging him.

"Oh baaaby…" he maneuvers to hold my face in his hands and proceeds to plant his mouth on mine. His breath, thick, is vaguely tinged with smoke. I struggle with wanting to immediately drop to the ground and fuck him until I can't see straight. As much as I want to be free sexually, there are old tapes playing in my head saying it's not ok to "throw it around" whenever you want. Then I remember someone once reflecting back to me that I get to know men by sleeping with them. I read people through their bodies and their sexing. It's a language I speak fluently and I find comfort in the discomfort of not knowing its rules of grammar or punctuation.

My hand wanders to his ass—small and slightly softer with age. He unlocks his lips from mine, looks me in the eyes and caresses my cheeks with his thumbs.

"How are you sweetheart?"

We settle into a cozy corner table and become two of the seven customers in the restaurant. He orders us a bottle of red wine. He asks me what I like to eat, what flavors entice me. Perusing the menu, he takes my answers into consideration and orders for me. Perfectly old school. I love that. I feel cared for when a man takes control. When his control is rooted in service of my pleasure and his willingness to provide it. At a deep energetic level, it creates room for me to relax into my feminine soft place. The place where I want to spread open wide, take the man in, and give him my gifts.

We eat, drink and talk for a few hours. Our bodies touching each other the entire time. His thigh brushing against mine. His fingers stroking my hand, my forearm, my cheeks. He leans in to kiss me more times than I can remember. Our lips taste of wine, garlic, and thick tomato sauce brushed with basil. My body, light and high from the drug of him, wants to hurl itself onto his lap, straddle his chair and ride him all night long. I settle for kneading his inner thigh while he feeds me with his epic fingers. They ooze creativity and sex. They are perfectly shaped from the knuckle all the way through to the nailbed. I want them inside me. I want him to stroke my G-spot the way he plays his bass guitar—with focus and fierce passion.

He pays the check, helps me into my coat, and opens the front door. We remain in our pheromone-induced bubble as we float the five blocks back to his apartment. We walk through the metal front door to the inner concrete courtyard to the back building where he opens the next front door and then guides me up the staircase three stories to his door. Déjà vu flutters across my skin and I am 17 all over again. Groovy lounge music steeps the air. I immediately fall into the beat, my body gyrating to the rhythm.

"Here baby, lemme take your coat."

"Mm. Thanks."

"And shed your shoes. I keep it simple here."

That he does. The apartment is sparse. Appropriately so for New York. A bed on the floor, a tv mounted on the opposite wall, a table in the kitchen, a desk with a computer, and 5 bass guitars hanging on the wall, all echo the place on MacDougal, minus the roommates. The lights are dim and he keeps them that way. He lights a candle. I barely notice. Wrapped up in the reality of standing barefoot in his apartment, knowing what we are about to do and feeling equally nervous and eager, I am dizzy. He must've sensed this because he comes over and kisses me. My mouth opens to his tongue—strong and soft. He parts lips with me only to take my shirt over my head. Continuing our oral exploration, he unbuttons my pants, dropping them to the floor. I gingerly step out of them. Standing in a black lace bra and panty set, I wonder if he likes what he sees. As his hands glide over my curves, I wonder if he likes what he is touching. He pulls off his white ribbed tank and slips off his jeans. I had forgotten about his tattoo. A bass clef adorning his upper left arm. It's simple and to the point, like him.

He steps back. His brown eyes fixate on me.

"Oh, baby. Look at you."

"Yeah?"

"You look just like you did when I met you. You're amazing."

I'm not sure I believe him but I drink in the compliment anyway.

He pulls me to him and folds both our bodies onto the bed. My milky white skin tangles with his sun-kissed flesh. Both of us are soft and smooth. We are in familiar waters yet it is fresh. Like kelp floating in the ocean, we sway into each other, stroking body parts, hands over hands. His hands adorn my breasts, his fingers pinch my nipples, our mouths are everywhere. His mouth covers every inch of my chest and torso, eventually winding its way down to my pussy. One long lion tongue lapping and I can't see straight. Lower back arching, my eyes roll back into my head.

"Oh fuck..." he giggles between my thighs. "I remember your taste. Fuck. You're amazing..." his voice trails off as his mouth resumes devouring me. Dripping orange blossom honey all over his face, I cum—ecstatically laughing the entire time. He slows his tongue, concentrating on my outer lips and nibbling my inner thigh. Hungry moans rip through me as I grab him by the hair, pulling his mouth onto mine. I have to kiss him. I have to have the cum he evoked in my mouth. And now, I have to taste him. I roll him onto his back and make my way to his cock, which is at full attention. I remember his cock to be big, but details of it have faded with the years. Now, with it in my mouth, I regain its texture. Its shape. The geography of its terrain. It's thick, long, and slightly tapered at the tip. I can't get the entire length of it in my mouth so I use my hand to grasp the base of his shaft. Sufficiently wet with saliva, I twist my hand up and down, matching the rhythm with my mouth. He stuffs his hand into my curly mane, grabbing a fistful of me from the root. This only makes me suck him harder and with more delight. He grabs at me again, this time pulling me on top of him. One hand in my hair and the other on his cock, he plunges himself into my teeming ocean. My eyes open wide as I stare down at him. Both hands in my hair now, he holds my gaze. Steady. Steady pounding. Bass. Bass. Bass. He moves his hands to my breasts. Those fingers caressing and tugging me make me hotter, wetter. Then they coax me lower on top of him. Mouth sucking the bud of my nipple, he commands them to pay attention as my lower body rocks on his fullness.

He sits up, still inside me. Chest to chest we hold each other up from our backs and breathe into one another. Nothing else moves. Perched on the pillar of his life, I cum again in subtle, rolling waves. He purrs in my ear, "Yes, baby. Yes. Just like that. Let it go." The well of gratitude swells up in me. *He's healing me again.* Being this alive and connected to a man in physical embrace is what I longed for and thought might never happen again. Not like this. Not where both of us were completely present, alive, and hungry for the other. The thousand-year-old tears attempt escape but are denied by more sexing. He elegantly slips me off his cock and places me on my side.

Entering me from behind, he fills me up in one sharp breath. He thrusts into me, rubs his groin against my ass and just as I think I'll be split into two, he thrusts again. Repeating this over and over, I have no choice but to completely and utterly fall open to him. He fucks me without excuse. He fucks me for all the years I didn't get fucked like this. He fucks me alive. He tells me over and over how good I feel. How he always remembers my breasts and craves them. He compliments me on my ability and willingness to be fucked by him. He is behind me using the cushion of my hips as handles to guide him in and out of my swollen cave. I can't see straight and I don't care. All I want is his cum. I want to see it and to taste it. I want every inch of him. I pull myself forward, releasing him from my lower lips. A simple turn around on my knees and his cock is between the lips of my mouth. He is so close and I work him. I send my back into a deep curve placing my ass higher in the air for his pleasure. My throat bears down on the tip of his cock as my hand lightly tugs at his balls. One finger curls onto the flesh just in front of his ass and that's it. He erupts like a volcano and I relish in every hot drop. He roars and shudders, all of it spilling into a fantastic sweet laugh. We collapse into a sticky sweat and fall into each other's grateful eyes.

He eventually gets up to bring us water.

"I'd say we still have it," I flirt, propping up on my elbows and taking a big gulp of hydration.

"Baby, you're amazing. I get so hard with you."

"Oh c'mon now. That's you... you're a stallion." I brush my fingers over the jade carving of a horse hanging from a leather cord he wears around his neck.

"Sweetheart, this flow doesn't happen with everyone. I'd say I usually have a functional hard-on."

"Functional? Well, lucky me then because you could knock down brick walls with what you brought me. God, you get so fucking hard—it turns me on."

That's it. He's up and ready to go again. And I want him still. I want him and I want what we are creating in the now nighttime of his apartment. I want it to be the seed that birthed my re-claimed sexing. The seed that plants a fresh page in the story of my life. The one that knocks me alive again. I think that if I take him in until I literally can't stand it anymore then I will shake free the old demons. He and I will fuck them right out of me and open a space for fertile bliss to run itself rampant over me. A space created of pure joy and pleasure. This will become the new normal.

He has me from every angle and I feel the psychic sediment shake loose. I know something has cracked open in him too. He moans his pleasure to me. He mutters words—"I feel you." "So good." "Taking me." He needs to know there is a woman who wants to be lost in him. We sex ourselves sense-full. Hours and hours go by until we dissolve into sleep. Our bodies contort into a Picasso painting on the canvas of his bed.

We physically part ways in the morning. A fullness wells up in-side me. The co-created energetic blueprint of pure life force newly imprinted on my body and soul provide me with a fresh lens for being. The city, brisk, has a sparkle to it as I walk to-wards the subway. I take the orange line, the F train, downtown and into the day. I know nothing is the same and everything is different.

YOUR TURN

Life Force Center

The Life Force Center. Here lies the seat of all creation—call it chi, ki, life force, or Mojo. The rhythmic flow of the universe rooted in power lives here. Its physical location is exactly below the navel and above the pubic bone, spanning from the front of the body all the way to the back. A space perfectly brazen and bold when unleashed. Eroticism, sensuality, awe, and enthusiasm are accessed from this place.

Welcome to the pleasure domain of cervical play.

Your cervix. The long forgotten, only consciously touched during your annual PAP smear, pleasure point. It's not a spot that's considered on a regular basis. It's time to shift that.

The cervix is the opening to life.

It is the portal you come through when leaving the womb to enter back into a life.

It is the doorway that releases your blood every month for nearly forty years (from puberty to menopause).

It is the seat of your power center, which contains your life force.

The cervix is a BIG DEAL.

The light side of it is incredibly potent and offers you a world beyond your wildest dreams of erotic joy and depth of feeling.

The shadow side is equally intense.

The cervix can take a beating. I mean, what else can stand at the back of a room, take endless poundings, self-regulate, open and close when necessary, and protect the royal chamber? Nothing! Your cervix is quite literally a gem.

> **Note:** If your cervix has been removed, no worries. Focus on the ENERGY of the space where your cervix would be. Consider it similar to amputees who often feel their "phantom" limb. The energy of the once physical part continues to be resonant with your body.

The possibility of an open, juicy cervix is yours to create. It offers you the kind of orgasm that leaves you fluffed out and dancing around the house without a care in the world for days after. Like many things worth having, this magical spot can at first be elusive and downright ornery.

Let's be clear. Too many women have experienced some kind of trauma or sexual abuse. And the fact of the matter is IF the experience(s) has yet to be processed through the body, you will most likely have layers of energetic residue covering over your cervix. It learned to build quite a potent psychic wall (and rightly so), but now that you're here—ready to embrace and own your erotic nature, the walls must come down.

I know. I know.

Demolition and renovation are never the first things on our list labeled: Oh Squeeee! So much fun! Hear me out. You're reading this right now. By default, that means there's some part of you, however teeny or giant, ready to transcend the layers of protection. You have become accustomed to their presence and know they served you well. I get it. It's much easier to stay self-sequestered in a bubble of protection. What I also know is that what's waiting for you on the other side is unknowable until you willingly, vulnerably and playfully stretch across the invisible boundary and allow yourself to embody a new experience.

The tools and practices in this section are here to assist you with dropping the walls in order to burst into full capacity with your Mojo life force. Because when you do, the amount of pure power, pleasure, and pussy freedom is endless.

OK. Let's get your pussy purring, meowing, and ready to roar!

Spirit Tools:

The following items can transform and awaken the Life Force Center. Use them prior to your practice to set the tone. You increase your spiritual sexual connection by combining these spirit tools with the sex ones listed below.

◊ Anointing with Essential Oils

This is the practice of smearing or rubbing your body with a substance to bless and consecrate your body as a sacred, energetic space. It connects the physical with the spiritual. It's most typically done with essential oils.

> REMEMBER: Use a carrier oil if you have sensitive skin.
> Almond, coconut, jojoba, olive oils are all good choices. You
> use a few drops of the essential oil with the carrier oil to make it
> easier on your skin and still reap the benefits.

Life Force Center: Dot or rub the space between the bottom of your navel and the top of your pubic bone. This is the surface level of your Life Force center. It spans the area from the front of your body to the back and the entire breadth between your hips.

Oils to use*:
- Ylang Ylang (relaxing, sensual)
- Sandalwood (integrates spiritual energies, activates creative flow)
- Clary Sage (grounding, stimulating, euphoric)
- Cinnamon (healing, protection, oxytocin enhancing)

Elevating the Vibration with Crystals

Using crystals (forms of minerals from the earth) is as ancient of a practice as the early Egyptians applying perfume oils for health and wellness. Have the crystals in the room where you choose to practice, sitting near or on your body.

Crystals to use*:
- Carnelian (concentration, creative focus, connection to beauty)
- Amber (confidence, success, joy)
- Moonstone (emotional richness, reception, balance with emotions and sensitivities)
- Snowflake Obsidian (inner clam, self-acceptance)
- Orange Calcite (vitality, creativity, spiritual Mojo)

Create the Mood with Music*

Music for these practices is meant to open and enliven you. Whatever you choose, be sure to keep that in mind and let your body flow.

Music to play:

* Strings. Those gorgeous stringed instruments. Violin, viola, cello, guitar, bass, sitar, harp are some that pluck and strum the life force center's sweet spot. Any kind of string dominant music that has a flowy effect and activates a carefree feeling is ideal. Choose songs, albums that let your emotions flow. If you're wanting to go au naturel, pull up tracks with birdsongs, running water, or fountains.

Sex Tools*:

The following items are where it's at to get your Life Force Center alive and kickin' through cervical play. I recommend practicing with them all, but not all at once. We don't want your pleasure hat to get blown off too soon. Each tool provides a specific nuanced sensation, thereby helping you reach a new threshold in your capacity for power and pleasure.

Lube

The almighty and brilliant tool for your sexual pleasure—LUBE! It's the jelly to the nutbutter. It's the cream to your perfect latte. It's the red lipstick to your little black dress. It. Must. Not. Be. Overlooked. And I dare anyone to plead the case where lube *isn't* a good idea with penetration. We *want* you to be slippery and wet. It feels good and makes all penetration much more pleasurable. It's better for your vulvar and vaginal health too (your lady tissue is a delicate matter after all)!

As noted before, please please please be mindful of the kind of lube you use as all lubes are not made the same. We want you and your lady parts to be healthy, Mojolicious, and thriving. Choose lubes free from toxins and any chemicals that might damage your palace of pleasure and power.

Dildo

Merriam-Webster's definition of a dildo is *an object resembling a penis used for sexual stimulation.* Just like the penis, dildos come in all shapes, sizes and colors. Think of a dildo as a shaft of your choosing to worship, awaken, and satisfy your life force center.

Choose one (or a few) that look pleasing to you, feels yummy in your hand, and has a comfortable weight. Many dildos are completely smooth from tip to base. Some have the shape of a shaft and head, ridges and all. Remember, this is an object that goes inside you. It's a good idea to make sure it's made of body safe, non-toxic materials. AND let's be clear, a dildo does not vibrate. Vibrators are their own category of sex toy. They can be wonderful and many people find oodles of *oh yes* using them. For the practices here, start with the dildo. It provides a direct, unadulterated experience. We are looking to form a long-term relationship with your cervix and there's something to be said for going slow vs. a torrid one-night stand.

Crystal Wands

Oh baby! This is where spirit and sex come together. Where energy and sex merge. Crystal wands are literally a rod made from a gemstone. They come in a wide variety of gemstone materials from clear quartz to rose quartz to onyx to amethyst and more. Each stone carries a particular vibration, which means you get to consciously choose the kind of energy to use when awakening your cervix. They are completely smooth, come in a variety of lengths and usually have a tapered end on one side. Originally these were sold as massage tools. Now, there are lots of folks who make and market them as sex toys. Shout out for progress!

Speculum (extra credit)

You may only be familiar with the idea of a speculum for your annual Pap smear. It is the instrument used to open your pussy wide enough to see your gorgeous cervix, which rests at the very back of your vaginal canal. Speculums are an instrument made from metal or plastic. And thanks to the wonder of the internet, you can find easy to use, disposable (or reusable if it's solely to use on you) versions. They even make ones with an LED light built right in. Very convenient!

✥Permission:

Give it to yourself.
It's underrated and makes a world of difference.
I am giving you permission right now.
You are worthy of owning your erotic nature.
Now claim it for yourself.
Say it aloud: *I AM worthy of owning my erotic nature.*

By saying these words, you are free to experiment and play with yourself, relish in your sexuality and connect it to your spiritual self. You are giving yourself a gift by doing so. When you flourish, everyone around you will as well.

SOLO PLAY:

MIND

Now is the time to pry open your mind and allow the idea of cervical play to melt into its nooks and crannies. Wherever you stand on cervical play, it is absolutely one of the most transformative sexual experiences. The fact that we are still in a physical spot low on the body gives it a raw, primal energy that brings an enormous amount of personal power and Mojo to the table of your life.

One of the things women tend to struggle with is standing firmly in that raw power. It's been deemed *unfeminine, bitchy, overbearing,* and even *threatening.* It also gets confused with an outdated version of being a feminist. Embracing your *feminine energies,* the entire gamut of them, is essentially, feminist. And tapping into your cervix opens the gateway to access all your power—including that raw power, which is absolutely feminine! Look at a momma lion protecting her cubs. Look to Goddesses like Kali, Durga, Artemis, Lilith, Sheila Na Gig, and Athena. All strong. All potent. All wildly erotic.

Connecting to your cervix brings out the Warrior Goddess within.

It is incredibly sexy.

Creating an active relationship with your cervix, energetically and physically, turns up the Mojo dial and puts it on an all-access life-time pass. You can turn it up or down at your leisure. And that capacity is incredibly attractive, not to mention, practical.

You might need to let go of the idea that the cervix:

- is a place of pain
- is only for a medical exam
- has no use for a healthy sex life
- is too difficult to reach
- or any other idea you've picked up

Give yourself the opportunity to get to know yourself; truly, madly, deeply. Get ready. Get set. Let's get cervical.

BODY

One thing that always sets your fierce feminine, and therefore your cervix, at ease is having clear boundaries. A container. The knowing that there is an A to B. A start and a stop. This kind of *energetic and practical* support sets the stage for successfully awakening your life force center through your cervix.

You can set this up by simply setting a timer for your self-pleasure practice. Or putting a date and time on your calendar to block it out on your schedule. Turning off your notifications on all digital devices helps set the tone. Heck, put your phone on airplane mode or go crazy and turn the whole thing OFF (wild concept, I know).

Claim this practice as sacred time with one, some or all of these suggested intentions. Say them aloud with as much Mojo as you can muster.

- ✦ It is safe to explore my erotic nature
- ✦ Being erotically alive feels good
- ✦ It's good to be erotically alive
- ✦ I am willing to go deep with my sexual expression
- ✦ I love being in touch with my cervix

✧ My cervix is a source of pure possibility and pleasure
✧ Releasing old thoughts and feelings associated with my cervix is easy and effortless
✧ When I feel my cervix, I feel my lifeforce
✧ I enjoy cultivating a relationship with my cervix

Next, make sure you have the suggested tools you want to use nearby.

Get into a comfortable position. This varies and needs to work with your particular body. You could be on your back with knees bent pointing to the ceiling. You could be on your side or on your belly. Find the position that enhances the moment, not one that's going to distract you.

Once you're cozy and ready, cup your vulva with your palm. Wrap your hand across the naked flesh of your vulva. Say *hello, pussy*. And breathe. Nice. Slow. Deep. Breaths.

Inhale hello. Exhale fear.
Inhale yes. Exhale shame.
Inhale opening. Exhale protection.

From here, get your lube and apply it to your vulva. Allow your hand to explore the area, warm her up like the morning sun pressing into the earth and making her dew all over herself. As you move your fingers around, you can stroke, pinch, massage, or anything else that feels good. You want your vulva to plump up, flush with feeling, and begin to crave more. You are prepping your pussy to desire penetration. Going slow is always recommended.

There's a moment I highly encourage you to become intensely familiar with—your pussy's green light for penetration. She is always clear with this. Never confused. Your mind is the part that slips in and makes counter-pussy decisions. The mind can be THE biggest cock blocker out there. When you are in the early stages of listening to her, take a beat each time you get a signal. Breathe. Make sure the green light is in fact emanating from down there.

Once you have the clarity and confidence it is your Lady P speaking, she will want to pull something inside. You can tangibly feel her hunger. Her primal nature begins to purr, sigh, and ache for fulfillment.

At this point, you have a choice. You can start with inserting your finger or you can use the sex toy of your choosing. Depending on the shape and length of the vaginal canal, your finger may or may not reach your cervix. It's worth a moment to explore digitally (the finger kind, wink wink) as this gives an up close and personal encounter with discovering the terrain of your cervix. Whether you use your finger or a sex toy, approach the cervix with reverence. Remember, she's like the crown topping your life force center (some people refer to her appearance as a beret, but I like to think of her as much more royal than that).

Gently move your chosen penetration tool in and out. Go at a slow pace. No jack hammering here. With each thrust, go a teeny bit deeper until you get to a "stopping point." The back end of your vaginal canal is the cervix. When you make contact, it might feel painful. Or uncomfortable. Or strange. Or irritating. OR it might feel delicious. If it's anything less than delicious, be patient. It will get there in time.

Now that you've made contact, lightly press your pleasure tool into the cervix to give it some pressure. Kind of like when you're on the couch with a cozy friend and your shoulder leans into them, physically saying, Hello. I'm here. Your cervix wants to get cozy with you. She wants to wake up. She craves aliveness. It's her natural state of being. Once you get her to accept and welcome the pressure, begin a subtle (and honey, I mean *subtle*) tapping motion into the cervix. Understated is the name of the game here so that you don't hurt yourself, because that will certainly kill the mood.

Tap, tap, tap.

Tap, tap, tap.

Tap, tap, tap.

Get into a steady rhythm. She may begin to bloom from this and you may find low, guttural moans or groans escape your mouth. Or you may feel her shudder with fear and tears well up in your eyes. Either way or whatever else between, *keep going*.

Lady Cervix needs to go the whole race. She's not a half marathon kind of gal. She. Wants. It. All. And she really doesn't like stopping even when everything in your mind is attempting to trick you into doing so. She wants to be obliterated in the best way. With love and consciousness. Give it to her. Give it to yourself.

Experiment with movement. Shift your body position if you need or want a mini break. Shift the rhythm of your penetration. Pull out for a few moments and rub your labia and clitoris reminding them they're important party guests and you didn't forget about them. But don't let them get too chatty and distract you from the honored guest. Go back to penetration and acknowledge your sweet, throbbing cervix.

Consider relaxing her. Intentionally put your attention on her. Place your mind's eye on her and see about letting her exhale to the point of spreading out. She may want to rub herself on the tip of your tool. She may want to grind on it. Give her a chance to move in the way *she* wants. Instead of you being the driver of penetration, turn the lead over to her. She knows how she wants to open. She knows how big her desire is for release and acknowledgment.

Again, at this point, you may be in a wet pool of tears or writhing in animalistic glee.

Let. Yourself. Go.

Give yourself the freedom to feel, experiment, transform and experience new layers of your erotic nature. Keep going with what brings you and your cervix alive.

You may be wondering: will I orgasm? And the answer is: maybe.

Cervical orgasms are incredibly intense (like, full body, shower of stars kind of delicious intense). They generally require an extraordinary amount of trust. Of yourself or a partner. Don't be upset if your cervix isn't prepared to offer up an O in the early stages. That's totally normal. Consider the beginning stages as orgasm training. Practice makes for the big O.

When a cervical orgasm does appear, she's like no other. She is the baddest bitch in the room. She takes no prisoners. She doesn't care who's looking. She struts her saucy self all over the damn place. And literally might be the origin of not giving a fuck. Why? Because she kicks, claws, writhes, reels, and sashays her way through you. No matter what. When she feels safe enough to come out, there's no wondering if she's there. You know it. And you are left splayed wide open. Could be in a pool of tears, laughter or most likely, a combo pack.

Solo practice is a potent way to enhance the relationship with your cervix and it primes the path for her being willing to stay open when a partner joins the picture. One thing that makes the world of difference with cervical play is *aftercare*.

When you're solo, this can look like:

* Gentle rocking side to side or back and forth
* Light stroking of your skin

- Wrapping your arms around yourself or any body part that feels good
- Curling up on one side with a cozy pillow or blanket
- Or anything else that feels good

When you're with a partner, this can look like:

- Spooning or being spooned
- Your partner stroking your hair
- Your partner acknowledging you in any way that feels good
- Sitting between your partner's legs and leaning your back into their chest with their arms around you
- Or whatever else feels good

In either scenario, it is a good idea to hydrate. When you explore deep realms of Lady Cervix, it activates your nervous system and could bring up those anxious feelings. Keeping your nervous system as smooth as a baby's ass is to your benefit. One great way to do that is hydrate. I am an advocate for electrolyte water, those added minerals really smooth those nerves and leave you gliding along.

You may also find that you are tired. As in, a deep, spiritual tiredness. That's totally cool. Rest. Let yourself crash out. It's another way for your nervous system to rebalance and integrate the experience.

Extra Credit Bonus Exercise:

This exercise is specifically to get a visual on your stunning Lady Cervix. While it's true we don't see our organs or the inner workings of these glorious bodies, there are some things too good to be hidden. Your cervix is one of those things.

I remember vividly the moment I saw mine. It was with the gynecologist I'd been going to for years. This year, for some unknown reason, she said, "Would you like to see your cervix?" I took a beat and said, "Sure! Yes! Absolutely!" She passed me a hand mirror and instructed me to sit up on the exam table. The task lamp was bent over blasting bright light towards my pussy. The speculum held her open wide and as the mirror angled just so, there she was! My cervix! So round. So glossy. So puckered and rouched. I couldn't get over her gorgeousness. I couldn't believe *that* was deep inside me and held the gateway to my life force center. Something shifted in me. It's like the moment Luke gets the power of the Force. Nothing can ever be the same—in the best way.

You are invited to have this experience. You can absolutely do it at your next gynecological exam or you can do it in the comfort of your own home. If you choose to do it at home, be sure to be gentle, go slow, and have the time set aside so you are not rushed.

The best way to do this is to set yourself up in front of a full-length mirror and have a large hand mirror at your side. Get yourself in the same position as your annual exam. Rest back, knees up and a bit wide with your booty scooted down towards the full-length mirror. Make sure the area is well lit and ideally, have some type of spotlight pointing directly at your lovely pussy. You can always use a strong flashlight in a pinch.

The next thing is to get your speculum. Lube is key (you're sensing a theme with it by now). You want to put enough on the speculum so that it slides in nice and easy. If you haven't read the instructions with your speculum, pause here and go do that. Get familiar with how it works *before* going all Indiana Jones and the Temple of Doom. OK. Now that you know how it works, you insert it and open the arms of it to the spread that is most palatable.

Sit up, get that light pointed at you and take a look. Isn't she AH-MAY-zing! I mean, helllllo?! Get a good look. Revel in her. Gawk. Even talk to her. Say hello. Recognize that you are starting a new level of relationship with her. One that's alive, conscious and committed to your erotic nature.

Once you feel complete, carefully remove the speculum and relax. You might want to write down a few thoughts. Journal for a moment. Mark this time as a line in the sand. The you before seeing Lady C and the you after. Notice what comes up and how you experience yourself in the days following.

SPIRIT*:

Sit in a quiet space where you can be undisturbed for five to fifteen minutes.

Light a candle if that inspires or feels good to you. An orange one symbolizes the Life Force Center. In addition to the candle, incorporate any of the additional spirit tools you are drawn to use for this meditation.

Gently close your eyes and begin by taking three deep belly breaths.

Let your low belly expand with your breath. Really stretch your belly out by how much breath you are receiving—as if you are pregnant with breath. Rest your palms on your low belly if this is useful to connect your consciousness to your body. Once you are connected to your body, imagine a small ball of energy, the size of a pea, begins to glow in your life force center. It gently flickers like the orange flame of a candle. It grows larger and brighter with each breath. As the illumination glows, you suddenly see the most gorgeous, expansive garden in your Life Force Center. It's wide open. Lush. Fertile. It smells alive and moist, like the embodiment of Mother Earth herself. The garden seems infinite with nothing but spaciousness. There's clear, open sky everywhere and land all around as far as you can see.

A warm, soft voice speaks from the ethers.

"What do you desire? Your desire is my pleasure. Tell me. Show me."

You notice a watering pot by your side. It's decorated with brightly colored gemstones that sparkle in the light. Instinctively, you pick it up and begin to walk around the garden pausing only when your Life Force Center feels a *pah-pow*! In that moment, you pour from the watering pot silently speaking the vision of your desire. Liquid sunlight spills onto the land and instantly your first desire blossoms to the surface like a hologram. It's vivid and shows a detailed picture of what you want to create. You marvel at the image and take a big deep belly breath, inhaling the reality of your desire so that it merges *in* you.

You continue moving through the garden and pause only when you feel the familiar *pah-pow* in your Life Force Center. Again, you pour from the watering pot and watch your next desire sprout to life. Breathe it in. Continue moving around your garden repeating this process until you feel complete.

Rest your watering pot down and observe all the desires you birthed across your garden. Notice how they sparkle and shine. Notice how they pulsate with pure creative life force. Notice how effortless they are—right there within your energy field. Take a deep breath in and out.

Suddenly you hear a gentle whooshing sound. Like a soft river calling you towards it. In the distance you see the familiar flicker of the orange flame and move towards it. As you move, you sense all your desires are going with you. You realize, they are in you.

The flame beckons and when you are standing right in front of it, you instinctively leap into it. One, two, three. Leap!

You and the flame are one. You burn brightly. Glowing like a fire opal. And just as the opal glitters, you see glittery embers flitting into the air. Each contains particles of your desires. They pass through your belly button, moving out from your Life Force Center and float into the air around you like fireflies. Your body is now surrounded with these sparkly particles and every pore of your skin pulses with Mojo. Sit in the experience for a few moments.

Now, Take a deep breath.
    In and out.
    And another.
    And one more.

Consciously open your belly button energetically and call back your desires. Let the crystalline particles weave, twirl, and make their way back to you through your Life Force Center. When you sense you are complete, close the doorway of your belly button and rest in the fullness within your Life Force Center. Notice any sensations there. Take a few moments to remerge with this energy.

When you are complete, take a deep belly breath, in and out, and slowly open your eyes.

Welcome back.

* *Visit www.undressedbook.com for your free downloadable resource lists and guided meditation*

CORE

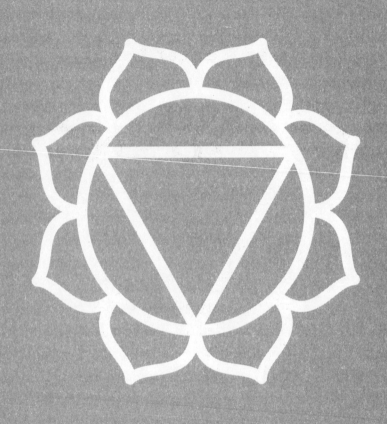

Power Center No. 3

CONFIDENCE

Color: **YELLOW**

Sense: **SIGHT**

Element: **FIRE**

Physical Location: **SOLAR PLEXUS**

{the area between your diaphragm and belly button}

Objective

The Confidence Center is the seat of your courage, determination, and ambition. This is where you experience your sense of self. This center gives you the strength of transformation. Here you can turn dust into gold. Leadership, self-esteem, self-discipline, and self-reliance are all available here. This center contains your digestive fire to support you in assimilating life, relationships, and actual nutrition.

Harmony

You have energy, willpower, and initiative to go for your desires. There's a clear direction to your path. When a bump occurs, you swiftly readjust without taking it personally. Your feelings are an ally to inform you of your next steps. They are easily integrated. You are filled with light and radiate this life force confidently. You are a contribution to yourself and others.

Disharmony

Overextending yourself, people pleasing to a fault, and insecurity are signs your Confidence Center is imbalanced. Negative emotions of jealousy, bitterness, and resentment are also warning signals. You are manipulative and controlling. New and unusual experiences scare you and you prefer being secluded from life.

Non, Je Ne Regrette Rien

Everything's hot right now. The days are hot. The nights are hot. It's a slow fire that makes the air still and my skin sweat. I'm wondering what it is I'm doing with my life right now. Work is slow. I'm concerned about money. I'm worried that I have no worth in the world.

Traditionally, I allow my sense of self to come from the men in my life. Though you'd never really know that on the surface of things. I'm good at faking confidence. As an Aries, who are known for their bold, passionate, and fun personalities, I've got built-in Mojo that comes with the territory. Combine that with my Cancer Rising, typically known for its highly sensitive, emotional, and sometimes insecure nature, you get a surface that can be hard as nails with a soft tender belly underneath. You might not know it if you don't know me. Though, I fear the soft stuff is leaking out.

We've been dating for almost three weeks and now the whole situation with him is pushing something in me. I'm volunteering for the fund drive at the nonprofit where he worked when he first chatted me up. There I was at the snack table minding my own business when I heard his voice—solid, playful, and undeniably him. His voice is legendary in town because he does most of the voice overs for the radio ad spots in support of the organization. I turned and smiled at him. Our conversation quickly revealed we were both writers, performed at the same spoken word events even though we had yet to run into each other at them, and we both enjoyed good food. As we exchanged numbers under the guise of connecting to talk about writing, I hoped it was only that.

Much to my surprise, that first connection over a well-lit dinner and excellent food turned into a second connection that was an actual date. And then there was another and another. It happened like putting on a few pounds. You don't notice at first, but then you do and instead of griping and crash dieting, you settle into it.

We've spent the better part of the last two days together. One day we went around looking at dogs for him to adopt. It was sweet. I got to see his playful loving side. The next day we went sailing with his friends. It felt incredible to be on the ocean. Especially in this heat. There wasn't much sailing. More like anchoring. It didn't matter because I got to swim and frolic like a mermaid while the dolphins and seals romped nearby. We get along really well. He's very caring and considerate, making sure I am comfortable, sated, and happy. Me, I'm cautious of not coming on too strong, even though there's an invisible force pulling me towards him. I want to be right up next to him. I want to have him smashed up against me. I want to feel like a part of him.

I ask myself, why am I so attracted to this man who is over-weight, bald, and physically *and* emotionally scarred? Is it that he's unavailable? I have a history of finding men who are perfect-ly unavailable. Having had an unavailable father translated to homing in on the "unavailable man" vibration. It was imprinted on me as a child. As an adult, I am now aware of this pattern. I have zero interest in repeating it. I'm ready to slither out of that skin and create something profound, connected, and honest. I'm ready for something where I can be seen beyond the crusty psy-chosomatic childhood wounds, where I feel able to share the full-ness of *me*.

Leaving the boat on that perfect LA late summer evening, he walks me to my car. I'm primed and ready for a kiss. A real mouth open tongue swapping kiss. We have yet to do that with each other despite the fact that we've been on five dates. We chat at the driver's side door. No move is happening. I get in, slide the key into the ignition and turn toward the open door. With one hand resting on the door, he leans in and kisses me on the side of my lips.

"Talk to you later," he quips.

"Great," I smile.

To say that I'm confused is an understatement. Why doesn't this man want me? Why hasn't he kissed me yet? He can't be gay. Can he? More importantly, why is this bothering me so much? Have I burned my entire self-worth and confidence in life into my sexuality? This idea gives me pause. I know I'm more than my sex. But I know it in my head. I'm not sure it has migrated to my body, heart, and soul. I'm aware of my frustration. And I'm aware of his seeming nonchalance. Could it be his own cau-tion—a masculine shell of protection around his fears and concerns? Or is it him being push me–pull you? Passive aggressive? This man is giving me pretty clear signals he enjoys my company. He consistently asks me out. He seems titillated by me, but I'm not sure he is turned on by me. And that's a weird sensation. I've been asking for a deeper connection to a man but I don't want the depth to be vacant of the heat and passion two people can have for each other.

The tides turn the next time we go out. He greets me at his front door by taking my face in his hands and kissing me on the mouth. His brilliant blue eyes sparkle. I am candle wax melting from the heat of its own flame. I adore this simple gesture. My face in a man's hands. It brings out the feminine side in me. That soft underbelly willing to show itself. He has dinner prepared on the roof deck. The table is set with placemats, glasses, and a candle. It was thoughtful. Romantic even. An entire Middle Eastern spread lovingly resting on a platter. There are lots of small dishes filled with different colors and tastes. He opens a bottle of red wine. It's warm and pleasant, like our conversation. We eat and talk as the hot sun sinks into the ocean behind us and the downtown skyline burns brighter each minute. Nighttime city lights comfort me. That first glimmer and *whoosh*! A fire ignites in me. It can be in any city anywhere in the world. Magic hour is when I feel confident and safe.

During dinner the conversation turns to sex. I'm sure I bring it up. It's not unusual for me. I love to talk about sex. And well, this was when it all comes out. He told me he'd "abused" sex in his life. He spent six years in recovery for sex addiction and still works the program. He's done it *all* sexually. He's been working on changing his patterns. He is determined to have a healthy relationship with sex. He wants to do it differently now—slow. No fast moves. Sex got pushed to the last in line. Human connection stepped to the front.

I sit back and digest everything he dishes out. It's a lot. But I have a big appetite. The truth is on the table and it tastes good to me. Surprisingly, hearing him talk about his past experiences gets me hot. Sexual charge flushes my body. It isn't over the top, but definitely buzzing. There is a moment when I want to blurt out, "OK. Let's fuck now and get it over with!" Not a good idea. We've barely kissed and I am jumping to fucking? Am I picking up his sex addict persona by osmosis? Doubtful. What this tells me is that I open fast, like a brushfire, when given the right climate. Exposing of oneself, one's true self, is the right climate for me. Instead of opening my legs to this man in this moment, I choose to open my soul. Sharing my own wounds and sexual past. Our truth telling coats the table in a warm, sweet mist.

The rest of the night is foreplay. We go to a hip hop concert where he shows me more of his tender confidence. He walks with his arm around me, or at least guiding me, at all times. He is firm without being overbearing. These simple gestures, this way of relating to a man—or rather, a man relating to me, allows that soft part, the vulnerable strength of my woman-ness to emerge. I am the ground-hog testing the climate. Will I peek my head out? Will I see my shadow?

At one point the music is righteous, the crowd responsive, and he, nearly six feet and over two hundred pounds, stands behind me. His arm swoops around the front of my body, pulling me to him. The pressure of his hand on my belly and the sheer power of his energy surprises me. It is self-assured. Unapologetic.

Knowing. It turns me on. Each time I find myself doubting why I spend time with *this* man, he turns me on my heels. He is a clear sign for me to reconnect to my own power. There's no sense in second guessing all the time. It's self-abuse. I have the where-withal and knowledge of what's right and good. I believe that. The muscle merely atrophied. Being with him exercises it.

Back at his condo I am ripe for physical connection, yet prepared to drive myself home. I'm not interested in pushing anymore. The emotional and psychic intermingling with him satiates the old nagging need for proof of my worth in a physical way. I drink in his home. The bones are a stunning 1920s building, complete with crown moldings, hardwood floors, and spacious rooms. It's as if the building reflects what I desire to be. A proud, poised presence from the inside out. His furniture mixes form with function. Everything is deliberate. Everything has a sense of being. And everything is an accurate reflection of who I know him to be—stylish, with a pinch of sleek, and a dollop of substance. One large painting looms over the sofa. Thick brushstrokes form a Picasso-esque face. Draping down the edges of the canvas in big yellow letters it says: *BEAST.* This epitomizes the way I understand him. Challenging to look at for some, but rich with color, texture, contrast, and completely intriguing. A person's home is a reflection of who they are—I like this home and the person in it.

We make our way to the sofa. He pulls me close to him and pets my head. Knowing, without *really* knowing—he has me. I am a cat purring and prepared to lie on his burly chest all night long. I sense the little hairs all over my body stand up, excited from the attention. The brushfire catches a blast of air. His face moves close to mine. First, he nuzzles his cheek against mine—big cat to little. His mouth turns towards mine. I open to receive the moment. I don't open and push. I make sure I let this happen as opposed to directing it. His lips connect to mine. *Flush*. Heat licks my insides. The scruff of his beard rakes against my smooth skin. He takes one hand and places it around the side of my face, pulling it into him as he presses his tongue in my mouth. I am surprised how soft it is. How tender. It defies his outer image. I feel taken aback at how completely turned on I am to him in a way that goes deeper than skin. I want to crawl up into him and feel his pleasure. His pain. His joy. His despair. I don't want to fix it (my past reaction). I want to witness it. I want to give him the light that flows through me. No more. No less.

I spend the night with him. We do nothing sexual except kiss and lightly touch. I'm a big fan of cuddling and am pleased to find out he is too. It's easy for us. Our bodies have a natural magnetism. He moves one way, my body follows. I shift, he follows. We are doing bed ballet all night long.

I drive home early in the morning. Pulling onto the freeway, my ego snickers in the back seat. She is all sprawled out in a slinky leopard onesie, celebrity-sized sunglasses, and her signature lipstick; the perfect red.

"What?! What?!" I whine.

Ego glows a putrid sunshine yellow as she leans forward to wrap her arms around me like another seat belt.

"Don't be sweet with me," I try to wriggle myself loose. "And why do you always show up when I drive? Because I'm trapped? Damn."

Dahling, she purrs like Eartha Kitt, Let's be clear. *You need him to want you. You know that's how you're fed. It fuels you— and me. Look at me. I'm losing that happy glow.*

"You do look a bit washed out," I muster, half wanting to piss her off.

There's my girrrrl, she strokes my head, leans back, and fades into the rearview.

She's a familiar feeling, but not as comforting as I remembered. She feels bristly. Constricted. Kind of like I gained weight or she shrunk and we don't fit anymore. I keep that to myself for the moment. I am not ready to fight her off.

We continued to date, he and I. The heat of Summer faded into a nearly-as-hot early Fall. I continue to be soft and sweet while practicing being in the moment; something different for me. The Italians say, "Piano, piano" (pronounced pee-ah-no, pee-ah-no). Meaning slowly, slowly. No rush. Take your time.

Sitting at my desk post yoga, dinner, and shower, the computer has me locked in its glow-y trance. There is nothing of importance. I'm going through emails, mapping out the week's schedule, and listening to music. The phone rings. It's him. He's been on my mind a lot this week and I am glad he tuned in.

"Are you open to having company tonight?" he asks.

"Sure," I reply.

"Yeah. I don't feel like sleeping alone," he trails off.

I've been wanting to have another sleep over with him. His passion for life, food, drugs, drink, art, and sex keeps me coming back. That and I love the way he touches me. Holds me. He seems like he wants to wrap himself around, in, over, and through me. Maybe it's that feeling of being claimed. Or maybe it is the echo of his addiction. Or maybe it's me getting lost in a man. So much of me wants to be swallowed up and eaten by a man. To feel consumed. I feel like that with him. His utter comfort in himself spills over to me. It feels ok, more than ok, to be unfiltered and genuine with him. I love his kisses. The way his hands glide across my skin. I feel like a woman in his presence. I am unafraid to *be* a woman with him. Specifically, the woman I know myself to be. She continues to ascend from the underground of my Soul in his presence—all the more reason why he enchants me.

Snuggled up in the bed and asleep, I dream about sucking his fingers when I wake up to find him caressing me. Kissing me. And like the first burst of campfire heat, we are in the throes of it. My body wakes up despite its slumber. I feel the warm rush of sizzle shoot through me. I want his fingers in me. I think I might cum but don't quite want to.

He half moans, half whines, "I want to lick your vagina."

This phrase, accurate as it may be, strikes me as odd. My head gets caught up in the way he says it and I felt the division of head from body. He goes down on me. My head throws punches. *You sure you smell ok?* My self-esteem takes the punch. Thwack! *You might not taste very good.* My confidence shrivels up. Thwack, thwack! *What if he doesn't like the way you look. I mean, you don't exactly have a neat and tidy vulva. He could find it disgusting.* This uppercut splatters my Mojo onto the floor. My body rears her head and pulls my attention down to *his* head. Between my legs, he's hungry and eager. It is all a bit too fast for me at the moment. It sends my mind into overdrive, now doing doughnuts around and around in my brain. Do I want to cum? Yes. No. Uh oh. I am not sure. Around and around my mind goes. This moment, his hunger feels out of control. I don't feel like a part of what's happening. I feel like a fix. A dose of sex to satisfy his itch. With hesitant concern, I ask him to slow down a little. I want to see him. I want him to see me. Feel me. I want to *be* with him. I want to go *deep*. I want to be able to actually connect. The kind of connection where words are unnecessary and we can merge with one another and fade our individual hungers.

He kisses my inner thighs and makes his way up to my neck.

"Let's review the special places," he chimes.

These "special places" are his favorite curves of my body—the curve of my neck, small of my back, and side of my breast where it meets the ribs. He lingers in each of them with the precision of a surgeon. His tongue, fingertips, and nose are the scalpels. Cutting open age-old wounds to let the toxic pain and insecurity out, he sews me up with the overflowing assuredness of his body. The sultry exploration shifts into the comfort of our cuddling. At some point, we fall asleep.

I make tea the next morning when the bruiser living in my head gears up with hefty boxing gloves. Thwack! *You really suck at communicating in intimate scenarios.* "Hey! I'm learning. I'm practicing," I quip back. I feel unsteady and vulnerable. I call my dear friend. Always the voice of reason, she points out to me, "You've got this pattern. The day after you're with a man you beat yourself up and sink into weak vulnerability."

"Ugh. You're so right."

She continues, "Well, ask yourself what you'd tell me if I was going through this."

First, I have to ponder what this is about. Is it that I open, open, open and when it's connected to physical intimacy I go into judging mode, turning on the *I don't feel good about myself* meter and let it rack up a pricey ride? What *would* I say to my friend? It would be something like— "You've done nothing wrong. You're allowed to be with whomever you choose. Just notice how you feel with that person. Do you feel expansive or contracted? You simply need to let yourself be where you're comfortable. If it's consensual and you enjoy it, you're all good."

A few months later we are cozied up in a corner booth at Delancey, the new hip restaurant in Hollywood. They're famous for the pizza. Ours, topped with seared artichokes, roasted garlic, and perfectly gooey mozzarella resting on a crisp crust, is evoking *ohs* and *ahs* with each bite. Conversation is easy per usual, as are his hands on my body throughout the meal. His hand is on my thigh. My forearm. There is the occasional squeeze of my hip. And the always endearing brush of his fingers across my forehead to push away an unruly curl. Fancy sparkling rosé goes down as fast as the chefs spin dough by the wood burning oven. Call it a combination of the bubbles and many months of continued comfort with him, I blurt out, "What's it like dating me?"

"Mm. It's easy. Good," he mumbles with a mouthful of pizza.

"Too easy?" I chirp.

He washes down the pizza with a swig of rosé and thoughtfully places the glass down. I can tell he is pondering the question because he has that pursed lip, slight head tilt thing he does before sharing a carefully considered thought.

"No. Uh-unh. I feel accepted with you. And cared for. Never felt like that before."

I smile and cry. The tears are genuine and booze-filled.

"Thank you for giving me the chance to care for you... and for accepting it," I sniffle between words. Like the smack of garlic radiating from the kitchen, I realize this is the first time I considered someone before myself. The ease of simply *being* I experience with him allows me to practice being soft, strong, sexy, loving, and all woman.

His hand finds its way under my skirt at a red light. I am hot for him. Hungry. Food, drink, and open conversation is my ideal foreplay. I scooch down in the seat to provide easier access—the light turned green.

"Ok," he pats my pussy. "Put your vagina away. I need to drive."

Back at his place, we get naked and pile onto the bed. I am glad to be in his home. I need the change of scenery, plus I feel expansive in his space. It's literally larger than mine, but what fuels me is the fact that I can expand energetically here. We slurp, lick, and suck each other. Our bodies are the dessert that night. Sweat pools on both our brows. My skin is feral. His cock slips into me, assured and full of life. He pumps and primes me to take more. To take everything he gives.

My pussy inhales every thrust. She wants to hold him deep inside and grind. But he pulls out and leaves her momentarily whimpering.

Suddenly there's a small splash of lube in my ass. His fingers take charge, teasing and penetrating. The copious amounts of rosé and his matter-of-fact attitude disarms the normally in-place anal alarm system. I relax into it. And suddenly, there is *a lot* of lube in my ass. "Oh! Wait. We're really going to do this?" I quiver.

The topic of anal had come up at dinner. I'm not sure how we got around to it, nevertheless, it did and I had shared that I didn't have much experience in that arena. Only once and it had been fifteen years ago with a longtime boyfriend.

"Yeah," he huffs between heated breaths, "We're doing this."

"OK. Be nice," I coo.

He slides the tip inside while I lay on my back. The alarm system tries to arm itself. He hears it and stealthily shifts us, telling me to play with my pussy. I don't care about her right now. She feels like a distraction and oddly unhelpful. Now, on my side, he spoons up behind me.

"Take a deep breath," he instructs.

I audibly inhale.

"Good. Good," he praises. "Now, exhale slowly."

Like letting helium out of a balloon you didn't want to lose, I do as he says and up floats his cock into my ass. He moves slow.

"Breathe babe, keep breathing."

I do as he says. I relaxed. With each deep breath and subsequent relaxation, he rewards me. A small thrust. Almost delicate. Priming me further open with each one.

"Babe. I'm in your ass. It feels so good," he moans. "You ok?"

"Yeah. I'm good," I say. "Really good," slips out of my mouth surprisingly.

"I'm all the way inside you," he whispers in my ear.

Letting him have me in this way is not as much of a shock as I would've thought. I am happy giving him my ass. It feels like a gift we're giving each other. He is skilled, gentle, savvy, and takes his time. A true talent. The stark truth is—I feel safe with him. Safe enough to open like this. I don't have to hide or feel shame here. His full acceptance garners backstage access to *all* my parts.

We stick to each other in the damp sheets with deep cuddling all night long. In the morning, I feel different. Not the physical soreness. It's an opening in my sense of self. The comfort and confidence in my body, and with him, that allowed the experience to happen. His capacity to be himself, no matter what, no matter where, or with whom, was the training I actually needed. And I got it. More than the lesson in being-ness, it is the extra credit of self-acceptance. I don't need to hide anything—body, mind, or soul.

It was anal sex. It was nothing innovative, yet I am changed.

YOUR TURN

Confidence Center

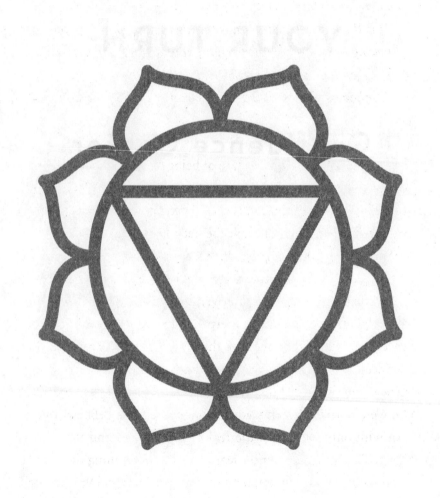

*The ability to be powerful in the world and feel safe in
one's body is the main characteristic of this center. This is
where you access the feeling that you matter in the world.
It is the place that generates the attitude of claiming you
belong here. Influence, strength, abundance, and wisdom
growing out of experience are all key themes. The
Confidence Center is where this energy lives in the body.*

Confidence. The elusive state of being. You think some people have it. Some people don't. And some fake it. Well m'dear, wherever you are on the confidence spectrum we're about to shatter the ceiling—no matter what the heck it's made of!

There are loads of confidence techniques out there and many people make a great living helping people access confidence. A quick Google search brings up over *eight hundred and sixty million results* for "confidence experts". What you're about to experience is the kind of confidence that's unshakable. The kind that lives deep in your cells. The kind that's connected to your very essence: your pussy. This confidence *is* your natural state of being. You were born with it. It's your Mojo power. It is believed we are born with only two fears: the fear of loud noises and the fear of falling. That's it! Every other fear you picked up along the way.

At some point early on, between the ages of 0 and 9, when you were most adaptable, open, and impressionable, you learned that certain things were "good" or "bad" about yourself and life. Naturally, the good became sources of strength, personal power, and confidence. The bad things became sources of pain, shame, and insecurity. You may or may not be aware of these things. The key is to become aware of them so that you can begin to transform them.

One of the main things we focus on in the Rock Your Mojo Mentorship program I created is how to move these restrictive beliefs out of your body. You'll hear me refer to them as kinks. Think of these kinks as the hardened calcified balls of energy (remember, everything IS energy) in your neurobiological structure that are jamming up your natural Mojo flow. This kind of *kink* doesn't refer to the sexual kind. That's another book entirely. These kinks, usually formed from some kind of upset, stress, or trauma experienced between the ages of zero and nine, are definitely in the way of your Confidence Center.

Here comes the antidote: Pussy Dance.

Get ready to dig in. Go deep. And get sassy.

By utilizing this new technique, you will gain VIP access to the Confidence Center and have her purring with potency.

Now don't get scared. This isn't some dance where you learn to twitch your labia and make the girls shimmy and shake (though that *would be* quite the spectacle!). This is all about you being brilliantly comfortable in the skin you're in. This is about you sourcing your confidence from the essence of your pussy. This is about you fine tuning your energy so that you are super clear when you are a FUCK YES! And when you are a FUCK NO! And responding in turn. This is about being yoked with your erotic nature, owning it because it's yours, and relishing in who you are.

Iris J. Stewart states in her book, *Sacred Woman, Sacred Dance: Awakening Spirituality through Movement and Ritual*, "Dancing is an elemental, eternal form of human expression, To dance, at its simplest, is to let the body express itself rhythmically.

It is believed we are born with only two fears: the fear of loud noises and the fear of falling. Movement, our first language, touches centers of our being beyond the reach of vocabularies of reason or coercion." She continues: "Dance is divinity, a natural state of grace in which we all reside. In its sacred form, dance is a language that reunites the body, soul, and mind. Working through the body, we integrate energetic information directly at the cellular level."[10]

This is why dance has been a part of the feminine experience since the beginning of time. We can see historical artifacts and references to women in sacred dance all the way back to ancient Greeks and Romans. It was a way to honor the Goddess and the Divine Feminine. Sacred dance is found throughout most cultures. It has been a revered expression of, and dedication to, *The Feminine*. The Pussy Dance practice allows us to tap into it.

You may feel confronted if this is your first time experiencing Pussy Dance. And that's a great thing! Any time confrontation shows up, it is an opportunity for transformation. Confrontation is a gift offering the reminder that a kink (or two, three, or a few dozen) is lingering in your body. You want these reminders. Without them, the kinks will hang out in stealth mode until some unattractive time, like when you're having the baum-chic-a-baum-baum with your lover and *PAH-POW!* Out comes the kink. You might freak out in any variety of ways, your lover has no clue what's happening, and suddenly there's a big ol' riff when you both thought you were having some simple sexy time. Kinks can activate in any circumstance. They don't give a crap what's going on. Claiming your erotic nature is one of the most potent ways to

---

10. Stewart, Iris J. Sacred Woman, *Sacred Dance: Awakening Spirituality through Movement and Ritual*. Inner Traditions, 2000. (pg. 5).

smooth out your kinks, tame them, and put them in the proverbial cosmic recycling bin.

You need to come face to face with yourself to Pussy Dance. You are literally naked in front of a mirror for this practice. It might appear that you are moving your whole body in a *normal* dance like way, but the truth is, you are taking all your dance cues from the *energy* of your pussy. You need to shift your perspective of who you think you are (ahem, you are a descendant of temple dancers). You need to be willing to accept the oh-so-Mojolicious you. Unabashedly. Courageously. Consciously.

Pussy Dancing ultimately enlivens you. It is incredibly simple as a technique. Once you let go and let your inner guru take over, you might find you never want to stop the dance because it feels so damn good.

Spirit Tools:

The following items can balance and invigorate the Confidence Center. Use them prior to your practice to set the tone. You increase your spiritual sexual connection by combining these spirit tools with the sex ones.

◌ Anointing with Essential Oils

This is the practice of smearing or rubbing your body with a substance to bless and consecrate your body as a sacred, energetic space. It connects the physical with the spiritual. It's most typically done with essential oils.

REMEMBER: Use a carrier oil if you have sensitive skin. Almond, coconut, jojoba, olive oils are all good choices. You use a few drops of the essential oil with the carrier oil to make it easier on your skin and still reap the benefits.

Confidence Center: Dot your midsection just under your diaphragm and all along the bottom edge of your ribs. Think of this anointing area as the area just below your bra line. Absolutely dot the front side, but you can take it all the way around to cover the sides and back too.

Oils to use*:
- Lavender (calming, relaxing)
- Rosemary (refreshing, active)
- Bergamot (strengthens self-confidence, self-assurance)
- Peppermint (reduces stress, increases energy)

Elevating the Vibration with Crystals

Using crystals (forms of minerals from the earth) is as ancient of a practice as using honey for its sweet smell and hydrating properties. Have the crystals in the room where you choose to practice, sitting next to you or placed on your body.

Crystals to use*:
- Calcite (removes stagnant energy, motivates, enhances trust of self)
- Citrine (overall wellbeing, security, trust, goal achievement)
- Topaz (greater consciousness, clarity, body strength)
- Tiger's Eye (inner + outer vision, sharpens the mind)

♪ Create the Mood with Music*

If you choose to play music during your practice, make sure it *opens* you up. You'll know if it does when the pores on your body seem as though they are plumping up—like when your cheeks flush after someone says that particular sweet, nasty something in your ear.

Music to play:
- There's a musician that has the classic sexy AF reputation every time they take the stage. Actually, it's two classifications of musicians. The reed and the horn players. Those scintillating saxophones, clarinets, trumpets, and trombones. Funk, blues, jazz, Latin, hip-hop, or orchestral genres are fabulous to stimulate the Confidence Center.

👄 Sex Tools*:

The following items are where it's at to get your Confidence Center alive and kickin' through Pussy Dance play. I recommend practicing with them all. In this practice, each tool aids the exploration and offers you a full-bodied opportunity to reach a new threshold in your capacity for erotic power and pleasure.

Clit Stimulant Oil

We want you feeling perked up for your Pussy Dance and pressing on your sweet doorbell is going to get you there. Why? One simple fact is that stimulating your clit moves your attention out of your head and into your lower body. Hallelujah and praise be! We need you OUT. OF. YOUR. HEAD. There are many clit stimulating oils. Choose one that's made of natural ingredients (your pussy thanks you in advance). Please remember, the nub tucked under her hood accessory is merely the tip of your clitoral complex. So, when you apply your oil spread it around on the tip as well as down around your inner and outer labia for full effect because your clitoral bulbs live under there.

Coconut Oil

Simple and straight to the point. Choose a clean, preferably organic coconut oil. You can find it at almost all grocery stores these days. Coconut oil has many uses from the kitchen to the bathroom to the bedroom. There's a full Mojo video I made in the Mojo Membership library along with loads of other useful content for your erotic and Mojo awakening. For this exercise I highly recommend you warm the coconut oil. The easiest way is to scoop some out into a bowl and microwave it. My favorite way is to use a massage candle that melts and warms the oil as it burns. This makes it easy to use for massage applications and gives it an extra cozy, sensual feel.

Robe

Let's start with all robes are not equal. For this exercise, do not use the super cozy robe that has one or two holes and a few stains on it. The one you sit around and binge watch Netflix wearing. No, no, no. The robe for this practice must be one that gives you the feeling of *being special*. Dare I say, regal. Dare I say, like a sexy mofo! Your version of this is different from mine and mine is different from your BFFs. Choose a robe that makes you want to wink at yourself.

Boa

Oh, those fluffy, feathery serpentine scarves. The boa. You might think of burlesque. Or stripping. And you are correct. Boas have been a signature accessory in both those worlds. It is time for you to bring one out to play with your Pussy Dance. Choose one (or some) that bring out the twinkle in your eye. They come in every color and a variety of fluffiness. Glitter or not. If you want to get uber-specific to enhance the Confidence Center, choose one in a gold, yellow, or ochre color.

Full Length Mirror

Basic or elaborate. The one requirement for your full-length mirror is that you can see the full length of yourself from head to tippy toes. Make sure it's in a spot that gives you enough room to easily move and enjoy your Pussy Dance.

✨ Permission:

This is your loving reminder to say YES.

Yes, you are allowed to experiment and explore your erotic nature.

Yes, you are allowed to feel and claim your erotic nature.

Yes, it is your birthright to connect your spirit and your sex.

You are worthy of owning your erotic nature.

Now claim it for yourself.

Say it aloud: *I AM worthy of owning my erotic nature.*

Give yourself permission to play. It's underrated and makes a world of difference. You give yourself a gift by doing so. When you rise and shine, everyone around you will as well.

SOLO PLAY:

MIND

Your Pussy Dance requires you to shake loose. This is a time to open up to the possibility that you are an erotic creature. That the skin you're in is stunning and your shape is divinely yours.

You may need to give up the thought that:

* Your body is a source of pain.
* Being naked is shameful.
* Admiring yourself in a mirror is vain.
* Expressing your sexual nature is dangerous.
* Touching your pussy is bad.

Or any other outdated idea keeping you from your most confident erotic self.

It takes a leap of faith to Pussy Dance and be with yourself in such an intimate, sacred manner. No one taught you this in school, but yahoo for you that you are here reading this book! I know you might be one of the six out of every ten women who simply do not look at themselves naked in a mirror. Ever. Or if you do, you aren't happy with what you see (according to a 2017 Women's Health Survey, 85 % of women didn't like themselves naked either). I know that the idea of not only looking at yourself naked, but *dancing naked* in front of a mirror seems as insane as bungee jumping off a cliff. This is where you get to set aside the mind chatter, take off the itty bitty shitty committee hat and tell yourself you will not die from the Pussy Dance (I really get it can *feel* that scary). Instead, you get to sweetly talk to yourself like you'd enroll a child into a new activity. This opens your mind and turns the confidence dial up.

BODY

Dim the lights.
Turn up the music.
Place the coconut oil and clit stimulant nearby.

Set the mood in any additional way that makes you feel safe, sexy, and a pinch silly (humor is always welcomed, especially when fear rises up).

It's always a good idea to state an intention. This grounds your practice and frames the energy with clarity and potency. Some suggested intentions for this practice are:

✧ I am grateful to align my pussy and power.
✧ I am willing to expand my confidence through my body.
✧ I am confident, sacred, and sexy.
✧ I see myself as a confident, vibrant woman.
✧ I am worthy of being confident.
✧ Confidence is my natural state of being.
✧ Being confident is sexy and I claim it now.

✧ Pussy confidence is natural and it's ok for me to have it.

✧ I love and honor my body in all the ways she moves and expresses herself.

Level I

Make sure you are in your robe when you're ready to begin. Naturally, naked underneath. You can start wearing the boa as well or have it nearby to play with during the practice. Stand in front of the full-length mirror and look at yourself. Pause. Really look. Look into your own eyes. Take a deep breath. Yes. One more deep breath. Continue looking in your eyes. And again, a deep breath releasing it with an audible sigh/moan.

Take a dab of the clit stimulator and apply it with love. If this is easy peasy for you, great. If it's challenging due to shame, fear or other concerns, it helps to gently cup your vulva first and say, *Hello, Pussy*. It's all about having a living, breathing, connected relationship with her. Once you say hello, you can slide your hand up and rub the clit stimulator over the sweet spot.

Continue observing yourself. Notice what thoughts or distractions arise (because, ahem, *they will*). Just as you watch clouds cruise the sky, let those thoughts and distractions float on by. Now, tune in to the music. Hear it as though every single pore of your body soaks it in. Slowly, without any force or supposition, notice where the energy in your body wants to move. You may feel a tingle in your toes or the tips of your fingers. If so, let them dance. You may feel a swirl in your belly. If so, let it undulate your middle. You may feel a bob in your neck. If so, let it rotate, stretch, and bounce. What's important is allowing your *energy* to lead the movement of your body. This form of dance is intensely subtle. It takes slowing down and being willing to get friendly with what's happening in the depths of your core.

Continue looking at your reflection. Follow your energy's lead. Most likely, your dance starts off slow. Possibly imperceptible movement. Once you tap in, allow the energy to grow in whatever way feels best. If you feel stuck, try something basic. Roll one shoulder up and back. Then the other. Then roll your rib cage around in a circle a few times. Roll it in the other direction a few times. Now, go back to rolling your shoulder and this time, peel your robe back and let it drop down your shoulder exposing your beautiful skin. Continue observing yourself in the mirror.

Let your body express, move, shake, roll, shimmy, glide, thrust in any and all ways that bring you freedom in your skin. Breathe deeply. Source your breath from your pussy. Let her purr you alive. Dance. Move. And drop your robe.

Yes.
You.
Naked.
Flesh.
Spirit.
Revel.
Bask.
Soak. You. In.

Continue your dance in the mirror. Wink at yourself. Smile at yourself. Blow a kiss at yourself.

This could be the first time seeing yourself naked and dancing. Or it's the bazillionth time. No matter which, make this moment count. Remember, you are doing the Pussy Dance. The dance where your pussy and body feel alive. The dance where you come face to face with yourself. The dance that ignites being confident in your own skin. The dance that reminds you who you really are.

Level II

Now that you're warmed up and robe free, it's time to take the Pussy Dance to the next level. Scoop a bit of the warmed coconut oil in your hand and begin to massage, rub, stroke it into your skin *as you continue the dance.* Your dance can be any which way that enlivens you. Standing. Rolling on the floor. Chair dance. Take this time to coat yourself in coconut oil, loving yourself up and moving your body. You may find your hands want to stop and caress your breasts. Or they might wander between your thighs. Beautiful! Rediscover all your parts.

Continue observing yourself in the mirror.

What do you see? *Who* do you see? Can you connect with the part of you that's beyond your flesh? The spirit part. The YOU part. As you touch your skin, slick with coconut oil, continuing to bring her alive, are you able to access the energy within? The energy that animates your being? You may want to close your eyes for a few moments to connect on this level. Once you do, slowly open your eyes again and do your best to maintain the connection with your spirit self as you dance, massage, and move.

When you feel complete, close out the practice by honoring yourself. This can be with blowing yourself kisses in the mirror, kissing your palms and placing the kisses on your body, bowing to yourself, or anything else that feels sacred and special.

As always, be kind and gentle with yourself. These practices are simple but they move a ton of energy and your system needs a moment to recalibrate to the new you.

SPIRIT*:

Sit in a quiet space where you can be undisturbed for five to fifteen minutes.

Light a candle if that inspires or feels good to you. A yellow one symbolizes the Confidence Center. In addition to the candle, incorporate any of the additional spirit tools you are drawn to use for this meditation.

Begin by taking three deep breaths. Let your ribs expand like an accordion with your breath. Feel your ribcage widen with each breath. Feel your energy sink into your body. When you are in—in your body, below the neck, imagine a light appears above you. The light has a color. It may be golden or any other color that evokes a warm feeling. It's gentle and cascades down all over your body. You are bathed in the warm golden light. It feels good. Safe. Comfortable. The light continues to wash over every inch of your skin from the crown of your head to the very tips of your toes. Covering you from front to back and side to side.

Take a deep breath.

Now, imagine the warm golden light enters your skin. Every single pore eagerly soaks it in. You get filled with this warm, golden light. You feel it fill your organs, tissues, bones, and muscles. Warm. Golden. Light.

This light permeates every single part of you. It is now your inner glow. You feel satiated with this warm, golden light. It gives you a sense of home. Your own space. A place that is all yours to create and live as you wish.

Take a deep breath.

Now, visualize all the warm, golden light filling you pulls in and makes its way to the spot in your mid body, just under your diaphragm where your ribs meet. The warm, golden light condenses itself in this area—your Confidence Center. It becomes a strong, potent ball of light. Because of its power, you may feel a pulsing or tingling in your Confidence Center as it coalesces.

When you've gathered all the light to your Confidence Center, begin to imagine the version of yourself that can do anything. The version of yourself that goes for what she wants. The version of yourself that is bold, proud, and lives out loud. See this version of yourself. What is she wearing? Who is she with? What is she doing? How does she feel? Take a few moments to anchor this vision of yourself in your body.

Now that you feel the connection with this version of yourself, let the warm, golden light containing the essence of her begin to shine out from your Confidence Center. The golden light beams out in all directions—to the front, back, side to side, and up and down. The light is so strong, so bright, so brilliant that you begin to melt into the light. Your body dissolves into the light until there is only bright, golden light. Your body is gone, the room around you dissolves. You are pure golden light melding into the golden light that cascaded down on you when you began this journey. Allow yourself to experience the sensation of being this expansive. This bright. This brilliant. Pure radiance. Rest in this sensation now.

When you feel complete, take three deep breaths to anchor in the practice.

And slowly open your eyes.

Welcome back.

* *Visit www.undressedbook.com for your free downloadable resource lists and guided meditation*

HEART

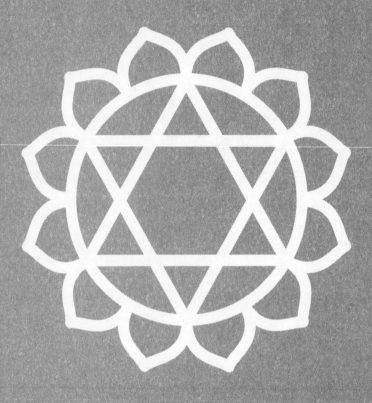

Power Center No. 4

LOVE

Color: **GREEN**

Sense: **TOUCH**

Element: **AIR**

Physical Location: **HEART SPACE**

{the area in the middle of your chest}

Objective

The Love Center is the middle of all the centers. It links the lower, more emotional and physical centers with the upper, more mental and spiritual centers. This is where universal love exists. It's been said that when this center is open and fully functioning, it has the capacity to offer spontaneous healing or immediate transformation to others. This center gives you a compassionate nature and ability to express unselfish love.

Harmony

You are comfortable with yourself and your perfectly imperfect nature. There's a positive outlook on life, even when challenges arise because you treat them as opportunities for growth. There's a natural warmth and genuine happiness about you. You form win/win/win relationships and connections with others. Seeing the Divine in everything is a daily occurrence.

Disharmony

Your Love Center is off when the majority of your relationships are toxic. You will feel uncomfortable being vulnerable to the point that being sweet or tender is off-putting. You have a tough time receiving. Sorrow and grief dominate your emotional state. You tend to be passive aggressive and it's difficult to get your needs met.

Lips Like Sugar

I wonder if this craving for claiming is lust for love disguised. Yes, love permeates all. Somehow, I've known this my whole life. I walked around, through, and next to love for years without stepping into it. Or rather, letting it flood all of me. I have an unwavering sense of faith, which is a precious jewel. I often wonder if I asked to have this faith before I was born. Like I knew I'd need the extra assurance this time around. Love. It's not the same thing as being claimed. Love can coexist with the claiming but they are not a two-for-one special.

When we met at a friend's birthday party in Boston, we were instantly attracted and drawn to each other. He looked strong, solid—inside and out. His nearly six-foot frame was lean, clearly all muscle. Close-cropped brown hair matched his brown eyes and his pillow lips covered a mouth full of teeth with small spaces between them. There was a depth to him I couldn't quite put my finger on, but I knew there was more than just a sexy package standing there. He came over to talk to me. His voice was coated with a faint Israeli accent. He took my number and called the next day. We went to the movies—our own double feature of "A Shark's Tale" and "Ladder 49." He rubbed my feet the entire time with his tiger paw hands to keep me warm. We ate Thai food after the movies and after the Thai food we went back to his place and slept together. It was religious. He worshipped at the temple of my body. He massaged, kissed, licked, touched, pinched, and brought every cell alive. He took his time and he was unconcerned with reciprocation. And for what felt like the first time, I let myself receive; fully. The strangest thing happened, only I didn't recognize it right away. It would take a few months and what some people call "heartache" for it to be revealed.

I don't beat myself up about sleeping with him. I let myself have the experience as a gift. I was totally content letting it be what it was—a fabulous one-night stand; until he called. Every day for a week after that night. Something about his incessant calls, his velvet green voice, his genuine charm, consideration, and the still vivid memories of his stunning body suck me in. We live across the country from each other, yet we find ways to meet up over the months. Each encounter grows in its intensity—emotionally and physically. We can and do stare into each other's eyes for hours while lying in bed with his cock inside me. We don't even move most of the time. The sheer pleasure of being that close is the thrill. He tells me stories from his life. How he grew up in Israel, in a small coastal town, with a younger brother, and his parents, still married, have a good relationship. How he was in the army and excelled quickly through the ranks. How he never finished college. It wasn't interesting to him, especially after the army. How the "powers that be" called on him for special missions and invited him to an exclusive training program. How he opted to go into the program, but not until he took some time to travel and clear his head. How he decided to go to India.

"I felt drawn there," he says locking eyes with mine. "I learned about meditation, yoga... and love," he continues, glued to my eyes.

It is a perfection of opposites. This man, trained to defend and kill anything in less than a millisecond, is the same man who melts into the realm of sweet emotion. He genuinely straddles both these worlds. This is a large part of my attraction to him. I sense this duality and it satiates my need for dynamic living.

Early on in our brief love affair, we meet up in New York City. I am attending a seminar and remember being overwhelmed with distraction in the afternoon session. The speaker, a man I respected and generally admired, is a blur. The hundred plus other attendees are negligible. The generic conference room, with its boring chandeliers, dull carpeting, uncomfortable chairs, and stale air are dissolving around me. My mind is consumed with the clock reaching 5:30 p.m. And, at precisely that time, I gather my scattered pens and notebook, nodding goodbye to a few friends. I ride the elevator down one flight to the lobby with my heart spinning like a whirling dervish in my chest. *Breathe*, I tell myself. *Just breathe.* Something about seeing him unnerves me in the best way. And yet, I am totally aware that I want to come across as cool, confident, excited, but unfazed. My heart is exploding in confetti like New Year's Eve in Times Square and I try to act like it's not happening. Hilarious.

I expect him in the lobby as we had arranged, but I don't see him. Then, with what feels like a spotlight shining on my body, my eyes target the source. They are resting on him. There he is. We don't say a word. He walks right up to me and pulls me into an embrace. Chest to chest. Groin to groin. Not even a morsel of air separates us. He holds on to me, pressed right up against him, and we stand suspended in time.

"Mmmm..." he hums as I blissfully sigh.

I feel our individual energy link into our combined energy. As if the vibration of his vocal chords sends a message to connect us again. A soul command that takes less than a minute to be fulfilled. We are together. No effort. No trying. His body is strong and solid against mine. His hand holds my lower back and my breasts press deeper into his chest. My nose nuzzles into the crook of his neck, cool from the late October air. Without a word, he smiles at me and keeps his arm around my waist as he takes us to the street outside and into a cab.

We giggle in the back of the cab like high school kids stoned on a hormone-induced crush. We can't take our eyes off each other. Let alone our hands or mouths.

During the intervals in-between our encounters, I can feel something bubbling deep inside. The calcified bits are beginning to loosen their death grip. The light he pours into my life has such a fierce intensity to it that the heat renders me putty.

"You're face looks softer," my girlfriend intently notes as she looks through the pictures from my last visit with him.

"Yeah? It does, doesn't it?" I reply feeling my heart swell.

"He's enough of man, or masculine enough for you to actually relax."

Boom. She calls it. For years, I have operated with a masculine shell to my personality. Yes, I'm clearly a woman in body, mind, and spirit. But life's circumstances have ushered me into the boy's locker room, so to speak, and, ultimately, I've divorced myself from a true feminine essence early on. Therein lies the pain. The confusion. And the hardened heart. With him in my life, I begin to feel comfortable "being the girl." Not only does my outward appearance shift, my thoughts and actions follow suit. I no longer cling to being in charge all the time. I am more aware of my breath throughout the day. I don't feel so desperate for male attention wherever I go. I realize it's better to light up a room *for* everyone, than merely to suck an ego, surface level response *from* anyone in the room.

I let myself receive and I let myself get intimate without attachment to the outcome. Because, do I know that he isn't *the* man for me? Yes. Do I have a fantasy that he could be? Absolutely. It doesn't matter though. I am so clear on the fact that he and I have fallen into each other's orbits for bigger reasons than either one of us can conceive. Who am I to mess with destiny? Plus, I tend to go full throttle with whatever it is I do. I commit. Even when I have a hankering that I'll get bruised in the process. I have always felt it's better to get in the ring and get dirty than to stand in the bleachers and only talk about being in the ring.

I am committed to having a heart connection with him. Our love affair teaches me how to fuck through my heart. How to give head from my heart. How to lick and touch and suck with my heart. Chemistry is a powerful cupid. We have it for each other on overload. Deceptive at times, it's nonetheless a high-octane fuel, and when put in the right vehicle it can perform near miracles. He is the yang to my yin and vice versa.

We float out of the cab into our sparse, modern hotel room for the weekend. He looks around, intently scanning the space—the special forces part of him is always on duty. Then, he pulls me into his arms and kisses me. His tongue darts around my mouth more anxious than normal. Hungry. Urgent. Like me, he's obviously been waiting to devour and be devoured for quite some time. I giggle, moving my mouth away from his.

"Let me put on some music."

My iPod and travel speakers are set up on the desk. I scroll through to the world genre, his favorite, and press shuffle. My hands lean on the edge of the desk, ass tilted up and out. An invitation. He comes up behind me with his driven hands, wrapping them around my waist. His touch is outrageous. Bold yet soft. Strong yet sweet. Definitely confident without being overbearing. We undress each other purposefully. As each bit of skin is revealed to one another, our faces simultaneously light up. Silly smirks turn into 1000-watt smiles. If every pulsing pore on our flesh were balloons we could have floated all the way to the moon.

Naked and alive, he gently pushes me onto the bed. His lips, plump berries, kiss my feet and attentively travel up my limbs and linger in all the right places until he reaches my face. Our bodies, covered in silky skin, effortlessly breathe together. His breath leads the way for me to go deeper, take more in, and relax. The Hindus speak of a God named Shiva and a Goddess named Shakti. They are the quintessential masculine and feminine life force essences. One needs the other to exist. It's said that Shiva, a warrior, is an unmovable force. Like a sturdy rock formation, there is nothing that can knock him over. And because of his strength, he can penetrate the ocean of life with incredible depth. This deep immovable force is what makes room for Shakti, all the kinetic, dynamic energy, to roam freely. Shakti feels best when she is unrestricted and able to express herself moment to moment. This concept becomes a reality for me with him. His loving force infiltrates my system, setting me free.

Rivers run down the length of his biceps and they swell with him leaning on top of me. I relish in his body. In his essence. I am awed by his physique and prowess. He's definitely all man, but he has access to his inner feminine. He knows how to read the energy of my body. His mouth speaks kisses and whispers licks to every part of my body. It tastes each corner of my terrain. Finding my pussy, he laps at it for quite some time. His tongue tells me stories when it is between my legs. Hushed tones dance out of his mouth into my velvet box and find their way to my heart. I melt more intensely with each serpentine flick of his tongue. He tucks his hands underneath me and lifts my hips so he can luxuriate in my ass with his mouth. I love that he adores enjoying my ass. He adores it as much as the rest of me. It is a sweet reminder that the whole person is to be loved. Nothing left out. As I am swaddled in this joy, he turns me over, until I'm not quite on my stomach, continuing to eat me all the while. Then, he plunges his fingers in me, up and deep, rubbing my g-spot. Surges of energy bolt through my limbs until I break out into full on body quakes. He remains steady, pacing the activity and energy coursing between us.

Soon, he fills me with his cock. His legs of molten rock wrap around mine, containing me in a vice grip as I remain on my side. He has his way with me and I gloriously let him. His determined eyes speak silent prayers. I hear them and place my palm on the middle of his chest to answer. My other hand, whispers truth without words, and finds the small of his neck. There is nothing else but this. And it feels so good. My yoni, the sacred aspect of my pussy, is swallowing him. His perfect size, thick head, and lengthy shaft touch me with grace. We roll over and I am on top of him, rocking back and forth. I ride the waves of the deep mellow love crashing on our bed. There is something ancient about the two of us in this moment. As though we connect to a space where we can experience love for love's sake. It doesn't matter that our "relationship" is in its infant stage. The chemistry between us is spiritual, defying tangible place and time.

We sleep like magnets that night. Glued to each other. He turns or I do and the other follows. Even when we have our backs together, we are touching. Early morning creeps in the window and finds us spooning. Sweet, soft kisses play morning revelry on my shoulder. If it isn't for his glorious hard-on nudging my back, I would think I am still dreaming.

"Motek..." he whispers in my ear as his hand caresses my stomach. *Sweet*. That's what motek means in Hebrew.

"Yafa..." he continues to caress, moving up to my breasts. *Beautiful*.

"Ani rotze otach," he shifts his groin and plunges himself into my morning dew.

"You already have me," I giggle and gasp with glee.

We make dreamy love this morning. Tangled up in sheets, pillows, and comforters. The hotel room bed is our own private island. He braves the "outside" world first by prying himself away to go to the bathroom and to order breakfast from room service. Two steaming pots of hot water for green tea arrive with an assortment of muffins and breads. He takes the tray from the server at the door so I can relish the haze of our loving that still lingers in the bed. Looking at him move gives me such pleasure. He is stealthy, yet elegant. He makes sense to me. Like leaves growing green in the Spring. It's what happens. It takes no effort. It's simply what is. That's what it feels like being with him.

We spend the entire day in bed. Racking up a total of eighteen hours starting from the night before. He continues to make incredible love to me. Over and over and on and on. Yes, there is

some fucking, but it is—something else. In addition to our sexing, we take photos. Photos of body parts. Biceps. An eye. Lips.
Ass. Torsos. Hands. And even one of his gorgeous cock inside
my happy pussy. It is as if we can't get close enough. We want
to see everything about each other and have the proof to remember it was real. There is a precious quality to the art of our
photography. It is up close and personal. Oddly intimate and
refreshing.

Being with him lets me live with my arms outstretched and my eyes
wide open. He unlatches the lock on my heart. I want to rip it off
and break it into smithereens. Seeing myself through him, I recognize that a large part of me was ripe and ready for diving into love
headfirst. But there is also a small part of me hesitating, not sure I
am ready for it. Or maybe I am scared of it. "It" being a relationship. "It" being the fear of letting someone else down like I did
when I was married. "It" being responsible or accountable to
someone else. I am totally unsure about all of this. What compels
me forward is the whispering from my soul. Combining that with
the chemical reaction my whole being experiences when I simply
think about him and you get the undeniable force that draws me
to him.

There are conversations between us where he accuses me of
pushing him away. More conversations where he attempts to play
psychologist to my wellspring of erratic emotions that he taps into.
And even more conversations where he can't understand my need
for self-expression through writing, getting more tattoos, or bar-
ing my soul on stage with spoken word. Most of these talks happen over the phone. That makes us crazy. Not being able to look
into each other's eyes or touch one another. He loves to be near
me. To keep his hands on me at all times. It is almost as if to give

himself the reality check that I'd really be there and he'll really be there with me. I love this about him. So being separated by three thousand miles is insanely frustrating. Long distance can add mystery and intrigue, keeping things hot, but when it comes to the nitty gritty of a relationship, it just sucks.

Despite the fact that we had a picture perfect five day visit only a week before, something seeps into the stew and it stinks. Is it his fear of fully committing to us or mine? Or is this not what he wanted? I remember what the small voice in me said near the beginning of us—"He's not *the one.*" I want to beat that voice senseless. I want to tell that voice that it's crazy and it is trying to sabotage my first chance at something real. At something bigger than I ever imagined. Then, reality kicks in. Like Shakti knocking me upside the head.

Hey! As much as this man cracked you wide open, he is, in the same breath, keeping you closed to the world you're creating.

Harsh truth. At this point in my life I have vowed to never shrink myself for anyone or anything. I've spent too many years cloaked already. This is the beginning of my time to soar.

And so, we end our affair. What most people call devastating heartache settles into my entire body. I spend a solid three weeks crying. I even glue myself to the couch for a day or two at a time to do so. Life seems impossible. The pain of losing him radiates throughout every breath and step. But one day, I hear a familiar tone. It is my innate sense of faith. She swoops in and whispers, *Let this heartache break you open. Let it give you grace. Let your heart grow even bigger.* Slowly, ever so slowly, the pieces of me form anew. I gain perspective and realize that I wouldn't change a thing. He was a reflection of the love already inside *me.* I might have lost him in the conventional sense, but the love we created will always be present. Now, I can stay in the disposition of "I love you." The heartache called "him" broke me open. He was the medicine I needed to remember— love simply is.

YOUR TURN

Love Center

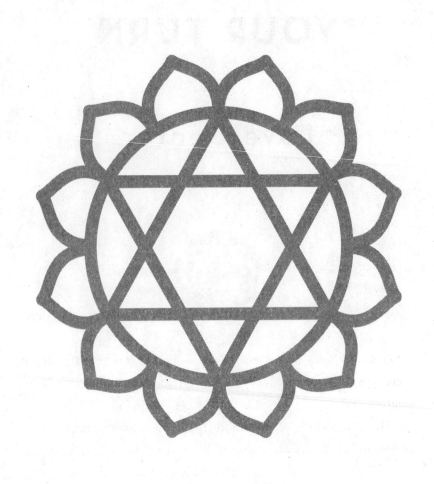

Pure love lives in the Love Center. The ability to be present and connect with another comes from this place. Openness, beauty, compassion, sincere involvement, devotion, and healing are natives of this center as well.

L ove.

Not the romantic kind.
Not the pheromone induced.
Not the Hollywood fantasy.

Pure love.
Unadulterated love.
Love—as in it's all around you, love.

We all want it. It's natural. The crazy thing is that we all forgot that we *are* love.

Not only are we love, we are loved. Period. So m'dear, hang in there with me because we are on a trip to activate your Love Center.

This is a good time to remind you of the universal principle, as above, so below. As within, so without. Basically, whatever is happening within you will happen outside of you. Yeah. I know this can be frustrating, especially when you aren't feeling so loving or Mojolicious inside. I promise you though, when you shift what's happening on your inner landscape your outer world shifts accordingly. It may be subtle. It's your job to notice. To allow the love that's always available to permeate your day to day.

Before we go any further, we must address the ever-present, looming ogre: the wall(s) around your heart. You, like most of us, probably have done some construction over the years and built a shack or fortress. You built it with good reason. Your heart got walloped, broken, and maybe even shattered. It made sense to put up protection, spackle the cracks, and install sturdy material that no one could get through. Deep security systems were wired in, no code was available to deactivate them. The issue with this is it prevents you from feeling, sharing, and experiencing love. Think about a lake near some locale that gets super cold in the Winter. Most of the year it's easy, calm water. Winter comes and that sucker freezes harder than the Hope Diamond. You know there's water under the surface, but if you wanted some? Sheesh! You would need intense machinery to cut through the hard ice. It's possible though not very inviting.

Your heart wants to love.
Your heart desires the juicy aliveness of love.
Your heart is more resilient than you know.

The freedom and power that comes from dismantling the walls around your heart is worth the journey to get there. Let's be clear: It is never ok to force yourself through this work. Take it at your pace. Learn your thresholds. Honor your nervous system. Regulate it to suit your evolution. Only you truly know what is best for you. Allow the voice within, your soul voice that speaks through your body, to be the one you hear. Let her be the dominant voice. She always guides you exactly where you *need* to be (which isn't always where you *want* to be, FYI).

How are we activating the Love Center you ask?

Nipple Play!

I can hear the oohs and ughs. Trust me. These practices are sourced from ancient tantric traditions, not a Cosmo article. Thousands of years ago, when women were revered and women's temples were the norm, sexual energy practices were cultivated and regularly taught. They were passed down through the generations and considered sacred.

Your nipples can bring you to heightened states of full body pleasure with their divine design. As Sheri Winston states in *Women's Anatomy of Arousal,* "[the breasts are] ... a luscious erogenous zone, conveniently hardwired by nerves and hormones into both the brain and the uterus." Your nipples are full of erectile tissue and when stimulated, they activate the genital sensory cortex. That's the same part of the brain that wakes the F up when you give love to your clitoris or pussy. Needless to say, we really are incredible creatures perfectly wired for the flow of eros.

Your Love Center rests smack in the middle of your breasts. Activating it through Nipple Play heightens the pleasure and possibility of love. The tools and practices in this section are here to burst your Love Center open so that you get to experience the love you desire.

OK. Let's get your nipples perked and ready to play!

{Love note}
Breasts. Boobs. Tatas. Titties. The home of your nipples. They get a lot of attention, not all of it *uplifting.* From puberty, to motherhood, to potential physical and health challenges, breasts can be a source of mental, emotional, and physical stress. If any of these are your experience, my suggestion is to keep the door open to your Love Center through the practices offered here. Experiment

with them in any way that speaks to you. And consider, no matter what your breasts and nipples have gone through, the energy, *your erotic energy*, is contained in every cell of your body. This is what you can engage. This is what's waiting for you. This is your invitation to claim it.

It may seem strange at first. This idea to focus only on your nipples and breasts. You may not even enjoy nipple and breast play with a partner. I invite you to experiment. Check it out. Choose this adventure. See where it leads. Be willing to greet a different side of yourself. Your erotic self. The you that craves aliveness. The you that aches for love. The you that desires depth. Allow those parts to rise up and lead.

These practices offer a new perspective on what love feels like moving through you *as you*. They open the doors to interact with life unencumbered. They become a portal for your desires to land in your life.

Ready?! Let's chip, chip, and nip away!

Spirit Tools:

The following items can balance and enhance the Love Center. Use them prior to your practice to set the tone. You increase your spiritual sexual connection by combining these spirit tools with the sex ones.

◌ Anointing with Essential oils

This is the practice of smearing or rubbing your body with a substance to bless and consecrate your body as a sacred, energetic space. It connects the physical with the spiritual. It's most typically done with essential oils.

> **REMEMBER:** Use a carrier oil if you have sensitive skin. Almond, coconut, jojoba, olive oils are all good choices. You use a few drops of the essential oil with the carrier oil to make it easier on your skin and still reap the benefits.

Love Center: Dot the space between your breasts. You can press your palm into this area and hold yourself for a moment when anointing. Your Love Center goes from the front of the body to the back. If you are able to reach the back of this center, add some oils there too.

Oils to use*:
* Rose (gentle, loving, transcendental refinement of sensual pleasure)
* Basil (courage, strength, purify)
* Myrrh (restorative, revitalizing, uplifting)

◈ Elevating the Vibration with Crystals

* Using crystals (forms of minerals from the earth) is as ancient of a practice as burning incense in holy spaces. Have the crystals in the room where you choose to practice, sitting next to you or placed on your body.

Crystals to use*:
* Jade (peace, harmony, wisdom)
* Malachite (confidence, transformation, breakthrough love)
* Peridot (light heartedness, universal love, free spirit)

- Rose Quartz (gentleness, tenderness, love)
- Watermelon Tourmaline (expansive, divine love)

Create the Mood with Music*

Remember, whatever you put on, make sure it opens and enlivens you. The music is an added sensual enhancement supporting you to open this center.

Music to play:
- Flute, woodwind, classical, new age, or anything that makes your heart connect with the "dance of life." Music can be as personal as your fingerprint. Always choose that which enlivens you, makes you feel deeply, and shakes loose the sediment within. You know it when you hear it because your entire body will hear the music.

Sex Tools*:

The following items are where it's at to get your Love Center plumped and perky through Nipple play. I recommend practicing with them all, but not all at once. We don't want your nips to wince and wither. Each tool provides a specific nuanced sensation, therefore helping you reach a new threshold in your capacity for love and pleasure.

Natural Massage Oil and/or Massage Oil Candle

Your nipples and your breasts are sacred ground. Make sure to choose your products with intention. You can use an oil specifically for massage. You can simply use coconut oil (remember, it's one of my fave multi-use products to have. Keep it in the bedroom, bathroom, and kitchen! We love a multi-tasking product.) You can get fancy and use a tantra massage oil.

The suggested essential oils can be added to the massage oil for additional oomph. If you opt for a massage oil candle (I adore these!), the same principles apply. Find one made from natural ingredients and be aware of the wick ingredients as well. The candle automatically warms the oil, which gives the practice added sensation. You can always warm your massage oil at home if you want to experiment. Ten seconds in the microwave does the trick. So does the classic double boiler method on your stove.

Feather Tickler

These are a must to have in your sex tool kit. They are often overlooked and labeled hokey. Don't be fooled. This little wonder helps you wake up to the world of subtle touch. For this practice it is best to have a small tickler. They come in a variety of sizes, however the long ones can be more challenging to use during Nipple Play.

Body Paint

There are a plethora of choices out there... thankfully, many are natural, vegan, and cruelty free. Remember, what goes *on* your body gets *in* your body. Choose wisely.

Nipple Clamps and/or Suckers

This isn't as scary as it may sound and if you have never used these before, great! If you have used them before, great! Like so many other sex toys in our modern day, there are loads of options. Choose a pair based on your experience. To really go for it, grab yourself a pair of clamps *and* suckers.

Mini Vibe

Again, loads of choices here. Though, most minis are single speed. I recommend getting one that has a variable speed to adjust to your desired level of stimulation. Consider one that feels good in your hand and is easy to hold. Material matters. Choose one that is compatible with oil.

Permission:

Give it to yourself.
It's underrated and makes a world of difference.
I am giving you permission right now.
You are worthy of owning your erotic nature.
Now claim it for yourself.
Say it aloud: *I AM worthy of owning my erotic nature.*

By saying these words you are free to experiment and play with yourself, relish in your sexuality and connect it to your spiritual self. You are giving yourself a gift by doing so and therefore, you are opening yourself as a gift to the world. When you flourish, everyone around you will as well.

SOLO PLAY:

MIND

Nipple Play requires you to touch yourself in a loving, pleasurable, erotic way. This may require dropping outdated shame about self-pleasure. You are here now. Reading this book. There is a part of you eager to bust through the layers of other people's beliefs to discover who you really are underneath it all: *an erotic creature.*

You might need to let go of the idea that your nipples and breasts:

- are shameful
- are only to be touched on your annual screening
- have no sensation or use for pleasure
- are only for feeding babies
- or any other idea you've picked up

BODY

It's time to bare those tatas.
This is your private topless situation.
Create the mood.

Maybe you swath yourself in a piece of silk, or a groovy robe, or a lace teddy. Get ready to make love to yourself through your nipples. Are you turned on by the lighting? Or does it need to be turned off? Are you set up in a room that inspires you? Is it igniting your sense of smell? Do you feel safe? Do you feel good (even a smidge?!). Yes? OK, good. It's critical to keep in mind that setting yourself up for success is crucial for having first rate experiences with all these practices. The more of a YES you are, the more you benefit. Your environment plays a big part in being a full-bodied YES—once you get in sync with it, you're ready to begin.

Claim this practice as sacred time with one, some, or all of these suggested intentions:

Say them aloud with as much Mojo as you can muster:

✧ I am an erotically alive woman
✧ I am safe in my body
✧ My body is allowed to experience pleasure
✧ I deserve the pleasure of love
✧ I am willing to love myself
✧ I am open to receiving and giving love
✧ It is safe to open up and experience True Love
✧ Love is within me and everywhere around me
✧ I am love. I am loving. I am loved

Level I

Have your feather tickler, massage oil, and/or oil candle within reach. These tools are your BFFs for the beginning practice... along with your hands (more on that in a moment). Now that you are settled in a spot that feels good to you—your bed, meditation cushion on the floor, a quiet private room—it's time to ground into your body.

Take three deep breaths.

Inhale... exhale.

Inhale... exhale.

One more, inhale... exhale.

Ahhhhhh. Yes.

This practice can be done with or without massage oil. I recommend you check it out both ways. Go for a dry run and then next
time use some oil. See which way makes your heart sing with *oh
yes!*

Take your hands and rub the palms together vigorously stimulating and igniting your Mojo life force energy. Your palms are
major energy receptors that give and receive. Ever notice how one
person's handshake can be such a turn off while someone else's
makes you warm in your panties? Energy transmission through
your palms, baby! It's actually one of the five keys to your storehouse of personal magnetism and a potent way to emit the love
vibes.

When you feel the warmth in your palms, place them on your
breasts with your nipples between the thumbs and index fingers.
Notice and soak in the warm sensation. Let your breath expand
as your hands press the sensation of love and aliveness into your
breasts. Let it feel good. This moment is all about you and your
sacred, sexy pleasure. Your love for yourself. Your erotic
nature.

Now, continuing to hold your breasts, move them up in the
direction of your chin, then out in the direction away from your
body (left breast goes to the left, right breast goes to the right) and
back to where you started. Essentially, you are rotating your
breasts in a circular motion to awaken them and reacquaint yourself to this type of pleasurable self-touch. Repeat this rotation nine
times. Nine is a sacred number. It is the highest single digit repre-
senting completion, manifestation, and tangible success. Obviously, with each rotation, do it slowly and with awareness—as if you
are touching the Goddess herself (because you *are* one).

Next, rub your fingertips together until they heat up. In the same circular motion as before, massage your nipples and areolae simultaneously with just the four fingers of each hand. You know how a cat kneads with its paws and looks like it's transported into sheer ecstasy? Consider that as you use your fingertips to love on your areolae and nipples as you massage them in a circular motion for nine rounds.

Time to recharge those fingertips. Rub them together again to stimulate the life force Mojo. When they are warm to your touch, use those love-filled four fingers of each hand and massage your whole breast in the same circular rotations. You guessed it. You do this for nine full rotations.

Once again, rub your palms together. Really dial up the heat here. Feel the warmth spreading in your palms like butter in a morning breakfast skillet. Once the palms are sufficiently saturated with your life force Mojo, take your nipples between your thumbs and index fingers. On an inhale, pinch and pull your nipples out slightly. On an exhale, release them. Repeat this nine times.

It's a good idea to sit in the afterglow of this practice. Slowly rock side to side or back and forth. You may find yourself rotating in small circles from the hips. Move the life force Mojo of your Love Center through your body. Consider picking up your feather tickler and caressing your skin. Brush the feathers across your chest. Brush the feathers like an energy traffic director moving the flow out towards your arms, down to your legs and feet, up your neck and head, and even down your back. Continue doing this until you feel full and lit up with love.

When you're complete, roll your shoulders back, shine your gorgeous Love Center out, and take three deep beautiful belly breaths.

Level II

Time to get your body paint. If you're not into the body paint or don't have any handy, lipstick is a great alternative here. This is the part of the practice where you create reverence for yourself and your nipples. You can do this practice on its own, however there's something extra special when you do it as a follow up to the Level I practice. Either way, be prepared to fall more deeply in love with yourself and let any calcified walls around your Love Center crumble.

Your breasts are the canvas. The paint will become the expression of your erotic nature. Before you begin, look at the paint colors. Feel from your Love Center which color resonates for you in this moment. Take some of that color and draw on your breast. Decorate and anoint your breasts as though they are sacred vessels. Give them the design, pattern, symbols, letters, or anything else that plumps them up. Consider you are a Great Warrior Goddess and the paint is your breastplate to be worn as a symbol of your love. Love of self. And love of all.

Let yourself be playful. Let yourself be free. Let yourself become familiar with this creative expression of your erotic nature.

When you are complete, take a deep breath. Go look at yourself in the mirror (if you aren't already in front of one). Admire yourself. Praise yourself. Love yourself. And if you're feeling a bit bold, and I sure hope you are, take a photo of yourself. Just for you. A reminder and symbol of your loving erotic nature and how you possess it.

Level III

This level of the practice is where you get to play with texture, pressure, and even a bit of discomfort. You'll want to be comfortable with the first two levels of practice before you engage in this one. Here is where you can find the proverbial pushing of your envelope to love. Your capacity to feel intensely while keeping your Love Center open. Your willingness to experience heightened sensation as an avenue for erotic nature to blossom. This is the level where you get to play with nipple clamps, vibes, and/or nipple suction toys.

All of the toy options here bring strong blood flow to the nipples resulting in hardened erectile tissue and increased feeling. Check them all out and decide which, if any, brings you to a new level of erotic experience. Nipple clamps generally come with the possibility of adjusting the gauge of the clamp. Start slow. Your nipples, like your sweet pussy, can be very sensitive and you certainly don't want them to screech in agony. We're going for another kind of screech. Similarly with the suction toys, you can experiment with the level of suction based on the product you choose. Placing the clamps or suckers at the base of the nipple brings one type of sensation and on the tip another. Which do you prefer? When you are ready to be a little *extra*—and I know if you've been working through the practices in the book so far, then you are open to being a bit extra—wear your nipple clamps or suckers and go make yourself a drink. Cup of tea. Splash of tequila over ice. Pick your fancy. Do it knowing you are a woman wearing nipple toys. Look at your naked chest with the clamps secured on your nipples. Does it make you smirk a little? Does it make your *pussy* smirk? Mm-hm. You're that erotic creature. Alive and well.

When you feel good and complete, be slow and gentle removing your nipple toys. It's best to take them off on an exhale breath. This allows you to retain the openness from the practice instead of clamping down. The only clamping we want here is the toy on your nipple. Once you have freed the nips, take a yummy deep breath. Let your chest swell in all directions, front, sides, and back. Now your Love Center is alive and kicking.

SPIRIT*:

Get into a comfortable seated position in a quiet space where you can be undisturbed for five to fifteen minutes.

Light a candle if that inspires or feels good to you. A green one symbolizes the Love Center. In addition to the candle, incorporate any of the additional spirit tools you are drawn to use for this meditation.

Gently close your eyes and begin with three deep breaths. With each one, as you feel the breath in your low belly, see if you can swell your upper chest at the top of the inhale. You may feel a slight widening in the center of your chest as this happens. Carry on with your natural breath.

Begin to imagine a low humming sound starting in the very center of your chest, inside your body. It's warm and soothing. The vibration begins to melt your heart. It feels good. It's as though your heart is a weary, overworked muscle. The hum massages it into bliss. Yes. This. This relaxation and softness spreads around the circumference of your chest. You feel your heart "smile." She's happy to be warming with you.

With this experience of openness and softness, you suddenly sense a pale rose colored glow, the size of a small gem, inside the center of your chest. It sparkles, like a distant star. As you enjoy the pale rose glow, a volume control dial appears in your mind's eye. It's a big round knob with the numbers one to ten surrounding it in a half circle. One is the farthest to the left and is the current level of the glow. You are allowed to take the dial and turn it to the right to increase the glow. As soon as you're ready, move the dial up a few notches, to three or four. Notice the sensation that occurs as you take the glow brighter. Can you sense your chest swelling? Or vibrating?

Take a deep breath.
Inhale. Exhale.

Now turn the dial up a few more notches to a five or six. Notice the brightness of your glow. She is starting to spill out and pour into your belly, neck, arms, and hands. She is vibrant, pulsing, and so very beautiful. Feel her embrace each and every cell she shines upon.

Take a deep breath.
Inhale. Exhale.

Now, if you are ready, continue turning the volume up. Go slowly with the increase. Watch the light grow as you go from six to seven on the dial. You go from seven to eight. Yes! Now, you continue from eight to nine. The glow is so full, so brilliant that she reaches all the way down your legs to the very tips of your toes and all the way up your neck, through your head and everywhere in between.

Take a deep breath.
Inhale. Exhale.

Now, you are ready to turn the dial to ten. *Click.* The glow is at maximum juicy radiance. She is so full, so bright that she cannot be contained to the surface of your skin. She begins to pour out from each and every one of your pores. Light rays emanate from within you generously reaching as far outside of you as you are willing to go. You may want to direct the pale rose light rays to certain people, places, or situations. You may simply want to enjoy the experience of being this glowing and vast.

Breathe it in.
Breathe it out.

When you feel complete with shining your love light out, now, all that bright, gorgeous light shines back upon you. Yes. The light shines down upon you. It is warm. Lush. Pure. This light pours back into each and every one of your pores. You are consumed in an avalanche of love light. Let yourself feel it. Let it shake loose what is no longer needed. Let this light break you open.

Breathe it in.
Exhale yesssssss!

In your own time, find the volume dial. You are now going to turn it to the left, lowering the volume from ten to nine. The love light reduces slightly. Nine to eight. A little bit more condensed. Now, eight to seven. Even lower at this moment. From seven to six and six to five. The love light is midway as it continues to shift from five to four. You keep slowly turning the dial. Now, from four to three. And three to two. The light is small and compressed as you now turn the volume dial to where it began. One.

Just like it started, the pale rose glow sparkles like a distant star in the center of your chest. You are conscious of it. You know she's in there. You know you can access the volume dial at any moment. You are safe with the knowledge that this love lives within and all around you. Rest in this sensation now.

When you feel complete, take three deep breaths to anchor in the practice.

And slowly open your eyes.

Welcome back.

* Visit www.undressedbook.com for your free downloadable resource lists and guided meditation

THROAT

Power Center No. 5

SELF

EXPRESSION

Color: **BLUE**

Sense: **HEARING**

Element: **ETHER**

Physical Location: **THROAT**

{the area in the front and back of your neck}

Objective

The Self Expression Center is the seat of all communication. It links your thoughts and feelings as well as being responsible for communicating the messages from all the other centers to the outer world. It is helping you to have deeper understanding of yourself and life. This center allows you to deeply listen and develop your creative abilities. You learn your inner voice through this center.

Harmony

This is when you easily and effortlessly express your thoughts, feelings, and emotions. You own and honor your communication, even when it reveals vulnerability or possible weakness. Your voice is fluid and pleasant. You are able to say "no" when you want and are not manipulated by other people's opinions. Creative expression comes clearly and you are able to express your truth in all situations.

Disharmony

You are intensely self-judgmental and do your best to conceal your true feelings. You speak without connection to your thoughts or feelings. There's a harsh quality to your voice. You tend to manipulate others. Expressing yourself is challenging and often makes you feel inadequate or fearful.

Woman in Chains

"I'm kidnapping you until 6 a.m. and then I'll take you home before I head to the airport."

Giggling to myself I reply with, "Oh. Well, OK then."

The world, well, the world with him is always according to him. And it is never as he says. For instance, he says we'll go out to dinner. Sushi. At the time of our midday phone call he isn't sure where we'll go—in the neighborhood or not. What do I think? I say I'm happy to leave that up to him, but I'd love it if he'd picks me up. I'll be ready at 8 p.m.

Meanwhile, I wander about my day, dealing with all the things that need to be accomplished. Really, I sleep walk. I am totally wrapped up in how to "handle" the situation with him. What strikes me the most is how difficult it is for me to access the truth of what I feel and then express it. It seems as though a chasm erupted in my soul—a long time ago, yet I had just discovered it. This is more painful to me than the pending loss of him. Yes, I feel alive when he and I are physically together. There's something beyond chemistry that entangles us. But it's only when we are physically in the same place. When we go about our individual lives, the tearing apart of this otherworldly bond dies for him. He is a bull killing me with his horns, piercing me through the chest, and pinning me to the stadium wall. Then I bleed blue blood all over myself until I am left with an empty shell.

He calls to say he is outside. Taking a deep breath and reminding myself I have permission to ask for what I need, I walk out to meet him. Per usual, all 5'6" of him swoops out from the driver's side of his midnight blue Porsche, full of charm and pretention, the kind true native Italians possess. "Ciao, principessa." A sincerely polite embrace lingers into the bond that forms each time we meet. He smells fresh. His hand on my low back is strong and I fall into him more. My fingers rustle through the thick of his black hair at the nape of his neck and I want to get lost in the moment. In this magic spell we have over each other. The one that makes me go mute and forget who I am.

We met a year ago. He, a short, dark, and handsome man, scooped me into his starlit orbit one evening at the local café. For some forgotten reason, I had a spring in my step that night. I waited at the counter for my tea to go and when I turned to walk away— *shazam!* He engaged me. His smile was like the moon when she returns to the sky; all crescent shaped after hiding in the dark for a few days. It was surprising, and totally refreshing at the same time. His hazel eyes sparkled confidence and enough mischief that they easily drew me in. Wearing dark blue slacks, a stunning white shirt with pale blue crosschecks (unbuttoned just enough), an elegant honey flecked sport coat, and caramel leather shoes gave him instant style cred on my street. Honestly, all of that combined with his accent got my motor purring.

In the midst of our banter I blurted out with a solid accent, "Sei Italiano?"

Admittedly, I get all wide-eyed and gooey around Italians. The Italian man persona was forever imprinted on me at the ripe age of sixteen when I had the privilege of living in Positano. I fell for and had an epic romance with a man eight years my senior and my neurobiology has never been the same. If I get even the teeniest whiff of Italian swarthy, accent, style, and swagger my knees momentarily buckle.

"Si." He brushed the question off and continued chatting in English, "... And I was just in Dallas working..."

"Da dove sei?" I was more interested in where he was from then where he'd just been.

"Lago di Como. Tu, parli Italiano?"

"Si. Un po."

"Ah, brava."

I liked to throw the little Italian I retained around whenever I could. With a *kah-pow*, it transports me to the country that gifted me with the life lesson of feeling free, sexy, and delicious in my body.

The first time I went to his apartment I found myself standing in front of his door in my good blue jeans, a basic black top, and stunning Italian leather mules. He invited me over for his famous risotto. I could smell it cooking when I arrived. Fireflies lit up my stomach, fluttering about nervously while an invisible force grasped my neck closing down my throat. I felt vulnerable, excited, and intimidated. He had taken me out three times before this— for drinks overlooking the Pacific, a blockbuster movie, and the

Klimt exhibit at LACMA with late afternoon tea afterwards. Each time, he had me held in his demonstrative beingness. I was mush. I lost my Moxie. I forgot how to speak up and pretended that I only wanted to be pleasing—feminine in the most powerless way. Say nothing. Be pleasing. Adjusting my shirt, I rang the doorbell.

Whoosh! The door opened fast, like a trap door on stage. One step and you're underground fumbling in the dark. The air heady with food and his presence gave me pause as I tried to find words. He took the lead, naturally.

"Bella. Bella. Allora." He kissed each cheek and took my hand ushering me into his lair.

"Here, lemme take your purse." He placed it next to the sleek modern excuse of a sofa. His apartment was sparse. A large flat screen TV adorned the wall across from the sofa. The only artwork were black and white photographs of naked women—very Helmut Newton-like shots. Body parts glistening with oil, a flash of light on skin, the rest were in shadow.

"How about a little Prosecco," he said, not so much a question as a statement.

"OK. Sure."

Standing in front of the sofa I saw the view. Mostly of the other building across the way, but from just so I caught a slice of the Pacific. The sun was already down by Malibu, making Santa Monica glow like tealight candles and the ocean glimmer diamonds. A psychological thriller loomed large on the flat screen TV adding more drama to the already Euro trashy seduction. I froze in time. Immoveable, quiet. An ice sculpture at the hotel buffet.

"Prego." His arm scooped my waist ushering me to the long white leather s-curve lounge chair. He placed me in the chair, the prosecco in my hand, and bent over me. His lips, warm buds, melting onto mine opened my mouth making the ice sculpture run liquid. I slid into the chair, he clasped my neck in his muscular hands and squared off face to face with me. A duel? No. A moment to show me who's the boss. Stay quiet lovely lady, you'll get fed.

He put the finishing touches on dinner—a plate of succulent tomato slices arranged like flower petals on a plate with a pile of Reggiano in the center. Crispy bread was warmed in the oven. And of course, his mama's famous risotto.

He escorted me the five feet to the small glass topped dining table and sat me down on the leather chair. Admiring the spread, I waited for him to get settled in his seat. He was dressed casually. Dark blue soft pants with an inky blue Italian athletic shirt. Two white stripes came from each collar bone out to his shoulders. He dug into the risotto with a firm forkful. I took this as a sign to start eating too. Delicately, I pierced the cumulous cloud surface, pulling up moist bits and placing them on my eager tongue. Creamy, rich earth, and decadence exploded in my mouth.

"Mm, buonissimo!" I complimented.

"You like, yeah. It's good." He replied staying glued to the TV still playing the film, "Have you seen this?"

"Yes. Funny though, I can't remember how it ends."

He didn't reply. Just kept shoveling food in his mouth while looking up every few moments to engage the film. I continued to eat. I figured it's the right thing to do. Plus, it was good. But I didn't understand why he invited me to dinner only to watch a movie and not speak to me. Say nothing. Be pleasing. Say nothing. This old-fashioned mantra chanted in the bowels of my brain.

After he decided dinner was through, he picked up the plates, took them to the kitchen, and then picked me up, taking me to the living room. Unsure of myself, I played puppet. Wherever he put me I'd go. Whatever he did, I'd do. My body open and eager to have him duked it out with my mind who punched and kicked him away. Again, he placed me on the s-curve chair, the cool leather against my back. He placed himself between my legs, his back to my chest. He watched the thriller, almost over on the flatscreen. His thick muscular hands massaged my calves. His back pressed against my pussy. I wondered why he hasn't kissed me yet. Or on any of our dates. I wanted to ask what he was waiting for but, my throat lost its ability to form words. Only my body spoke. I want you. But I want more than your physicality. I want *you*.

He reached for my hand and placed it on his chest. His pecs were perfectly pronounced. I caressed them over his shirt until I had to have his skin. Diving under the collar of his shirt, I fell into the forest on his chest. Thick hair covered his skin. Hair enough to tug, to run my fingers through, to get lost in. I'm a fan of chest hair. Bare chested men make me nervous. There's something too precious about it. Give me even a tuft. Just some semblance of hair to let me know you are in fact, a man.

My fingertips grazed his nipples. Sensitive to the touch, he shied away opting to snake himself around now chest to chest with me. His hazel eyes dug into me, his waist on the warmth between my jean covered pussy. Taking my head in his two hands, he pulled my face to his and kissed me. Deeply. His thick, wet tongue melted any semblance of the ice sculpture still standing. A moan slipped out of me. I grabbed his ass pushing my hot box up into his groin, which made him stop kissing me.

"Dai, dai…" he said taking me onto the floor. I let him explore my body. Hands unbuttoned my blouse, bra straps fell off my shoulder, lips inhaled my nipples, and fingers gingerly pinched them. I licked the length of his neck winding around to his throat. My entire mouth sucked it. I nursed myself on his throat. Maybe thinking I could glean the ability to find my speech through him. If I suck hard enough, I can take my power back. This oral sexing shot icy hot hooks into my loins. My body became dandelion whisps floating in the wind. Waves crashed through me as he peeled off my clothes. Bodies undulating, skin touching skin, our mouths found each other's sex. We spoke into each other. We breathed into each other. We inhaled each other. The wet dark waters of our lust clearly conversed, mutually agreeing upon cum. My pussy screamed—cumming, fluid and fierce in his mouth. His, salty sweet nectar draped on my chest.

That night left me physically fed from food and the fooling around. Though I was emotionally and spiritually starving. We danced around each other for another week or so, but I had to draw the line when he stood me up for a Friday night date. Literally, I got stood up. That was a first. And I hoped it would be a last because the aftermath of it was me, a puddle, on my couch for the entire weekend. How could I let this guy affect me so much and lose myself in the process? It wasn't the losing myself that was so devastating. It was the dumb mute I'd become that threw me sideways. He called incessantly for two days early the next week. I practically had to tie my hands behind my back to stop myself from answering the phone. He left fun sweet messages.

"Ciao principessa! Where are you? I'm thinking of you. Call me."

"Ciao bella! I'm going to the café. Are you around? Come and sit with me for a snack."

"Ciao angelo! Where are you. Come out and play. Call me."

All of the messages left me knotty and with a pitted stomach. I couldn't call him. He was the bad guy, right? I decided with the help of some friends to let this one go. No call back. No more energy given in his direction. Let it fade. It felt like I was coming off years of drug addiction, but I did it.

A few months went by. Life happened. And then *it* happened. I bumped into him at the café. I saw him first. I was at the counter paying and he was walking in from the side door from the patio. It was a perfect Santa Monica day—warm sunshine painting every surface and a pleasing ocean breeze whispering in the air. I felt the ice sculpture try to capture my body but instead I felt a brushfire blaze through me igniting my heart and loins. At that moment, his eyes met mine. He smiled the electric smile, though it seemed partially dimmed, as if he was waiting to see how I'd react. A force bigger than myself pushed me towards him.

"Ciiiaaao!" burst out of his mouth and then a kiss on each cheek.

"Ciao," I replied politely.

"Tutto bene?"

"Oh, si... si. Tu?"

"Certo. You look good."

"Thanks."

What did I want from him? To be something that he's not? That recipe for disappointment was one I learned and refused to repeat. You must remember that people tell you who they are early on. And then they show you. Trusting that has become terra firma. I needed consistent reinforcement of that lesson. The effervescent cheerleader for humanity that lives close to my consciousness' surface usually wants her say first.

"OK. I'm going to enjoy this perfect day," he chirps. "A little paradiso, no?"

"Yes."

"Ciao bella."

"Ciao."

As the months went by and I continued to live my life, there were more frequent moments of running into him at the café. Not weekly encounters, but monthly. Each one got easier for me. He was who he was. Italian. Charming. Sexy. I had to laugh a little. He was so on the nose. Like a caricature. I began to play back with him. Flirt a bit. It's only a game. He'd rub my shoulders as I sat in my chair. He'd interrupt me when I was sitting with a girlfriend and make comments about how fabulous I am. He'd say he's been thinking about me and we should get together. Get together?! Hm. The first time he said that I just giggled and gave him a look like— you've got to be kidding me, right?

"I've been wanting to talk to you. I, I know I didn't treat you well."

Seriously? Did that just come out of his mouth? Pinned to the ground in shock, all the while trying to act loose. Nonchalant.

"Let's get together. I want to talk to you," he said almost a plea.

"You've got my number," I chided.

The bigger part of me leapt out of my skin and stood stoic, like the first moment the genie pops out the bottle, and commanded, *No! I don't recommend this! Don't let him back in your life. You need to stand in your truth. You know how to speak your truth. It's as ancient as I. Don't forget.*

As soon as he walked away, I told my Higher Self, *"Yeah, he's got my number, but he'll never call. It's only a game for him. Relax."*

My Higher Self reluctantly sighed and dissipated into the din of the café.

A few more months went by. A few more sightings of him. Each one amazed me because whatever this intangible thing that drew me to him in the first place seemed indelible. His eyes lit up when they looked at me. In turn, mine blazed with desire. His smile ignited a steely sense of attraction. His touch, even just his hand on my waist when he'd lean in to kiss my cheek, relaxed all the muscles in my body.

It was almost a year to the day from when we first met that I found myself outside his apartment door again. We'd seen each other in the café that afternoon. A little chat during which the subject of my right shoulder and hip hurting me came up. It seemed as though they were out of alignment. He offered to give me a session, a physical therapy session. I completely forgot that he used to be a physical therapist and now, having a corporate fashion industry gig, only works on one or two A-list clients for fun.

"What are you doing later?" he commanded.

"Um. My friend is coming to meet me here in a few. But after that, I'm free."

"OK. Call me when you're done and then come over."

"OK."

I distractedly sat with my friend. I was all fidgety inside wondering what I was doing. Was I going over for the physical therapy? Or the "physical" therapy?

Standing outside his door, casually dressed, I mustered an outer layer of confidence. The trap door of his apartment opened and he cordially kissed each cheek. The apartment was dim. He took my hand and led me to his bedroom where the massage table awaited me with soft cotton sheets, the top neatly folded down.

"Prego, Bella. Take off your clothes. I'll be back in a minute."

It seemed weird to disrobe myself in his bedroom so clinically. Seeing myself in the mirrored closet doors, I looked fresh. Open. I was surprised how calm I felt. He came back in the room. Completely professional, completely controlled, he commenced his work. Those thick perfect paws of his poured an elixir of healing and, surprisingly, what felt like love through my body. I relaxed into each stroke, each tug, and especially each command. *Turn to your back. Breathe into your muscle here. Turn to your stomach. Press against my hand with all your strength.* I loosened, stretched, and forgot that he was a part-time enemy. At one point when I was on my back his hands, immersed in my shoulders, began their way to the center of my breastbone. Fingers concentrating on the flat space covering the exposed part of my heart. Breath expanded my chest. Is he going to cup my breasts? Do I want him too? As though he heard my question, he bent over me and placed his lips tenderly on my forehead.

"OK. Turn over. Slowly. Take your time."

I was in a massage haze. His hands worked their way from my feet, up my legs, to my glutes. You hardly ever get the pleasure of your glutes being worked on. It's a taboo spot in all the spas, but it's one of the most delicious places to be massaged. It also turns me on. My mind attempted to berate me for considering getting sexual with him, but my body and a coquettish part of my soul took the lead. His hands slid up my hamstrings, again stopping at my ass. His fingers worked into the muscle, kneading me open. With each passing moment I wanted his fingers to slip into the crack of my ass and down to my pussy, which was glistening with desire. And again, as if he heard me thinking his fingers found their way to my yearning. My knees dug into the massage table pressing up slightly giving him easier access.

"Oh," he sucked air in through his teeth. "Sei tutta bagnata."

I couldn't even speak, but yes, I knew how wet I was. He plunged his face into my ass, his hands under my hip bones guiding them up further to forage into my moist cave. He licked me with his perfectly able and hungry tongue. Darting into my ass as his fingers found their way inside my pussy. I moaned rapturously as he worked me to orgasm.

Still shuddering from the immense amount of energy ripping through me, he rolled me to my side. He placed his raging hard-on in my hands. I swallowed him whole. I wanted to hear him in my throat and ring out my ears. I tugged his balls with my free hand as he pumped himself in my eager mouth. I licked and sucked every inch of him. He held back his cum. He wanted this to last longer. He picked me up from the massage table and positioned me on his bed.

"I'm not going to fuck you," I panted. Fucking him was not on the menu. I could take all of him on me but not in me. That was crossing a line. And honestly not knowing what I wanted from him, I had to keep something for myself. I needed to declare my boundary. It was the beginning of finding my voice—as meek as it seemed.

"Dai, dai..." he implored.

"No. No fucking." I put my foot down.

He conceded by rolling me on top of him. I wouldn't put him in me, but I would rub myself all over his shaft laying against his stomach. I took his cock in my hand and used the tip to rub my clit. Already engorged from cum, my button pulsed faster and faster preparing to let loose again. He leaned up on his elbows to suck on my breasts. And just like that, with my nipple between his teeth and my clit on his cock we both came unabashedly all over him.

I woke up an hour later wrapped in his arms with no idea how we got to such an intimate embrace. A part of me wanted to stay, but the other part that said *take the reins and take yourself home* won.

"Prego, principessa…" he holds the car door open for me as I slide in. Eight o'clock on the nose. He walks around the back of the Porsche and hops in the driver's seat.

"OK. There's been a change of plans."

I laugh to myself. The world according to him. It's never as he says it will be. Always a last-minute switch.

"A few friends of mine are meeting a Chaya. I haven't seen them in a while. I thought we could have dinner with them."

I chuckle, "Yeah. Sure." Part of me is pleased. After the last few months of dating, actually dating each other—not just fucking, this is the first time he's invited me out with his friends. And as expected when dining with other Italian men, one of which is on a date with a new, very young woman, the conversation is surface at best. My Italian eats me up through his fingers all night long. Even when he flirts with the waitress his hands are all over me. Pinching my skin, rubbing my shoulders, massaging my hands, thighs, earlobes. What he lacks in verbal communication, he admirably makes up for with his physical talk. As much as I relish in him, the crisp fact that his unavailability is the most desirable factor, tears me up. With everything I feel for him, I can never have *him*.

I choose the game for this last night and play the pleasing role. Witnessing the stark unspoken truth that he's unable to hold his end of the conversation. And now, with my throat open and my heart in my words, I know it is time to let him go.

YOUR TURN

Self-Expression Center

*This is the Communication Center. Our deep truth and
total expression of self is accessible here. From this center,
one can find independence, inspiration, and access to the
subtler levels of being. There is a resonance of being that
vibrates from this place.*

It's time to transform centuries of repression.
We are about to radically shift the way you exist because, honey, if you have been shy to speak your mind in any aspect of your life, which is sadly the norm for most women, you are about to get the Mojo secret upgrade in communication.

Are you ready to have your mind (or rather, throat) blown open?! Here's a little-known fact:

Your throat and your cervix are connected. Yep. You read that right. The largest nerve, the vagus nerve, connects them. From the base of your neck to the pelvic girdle. And the vagus nerve is connected to the parasympathetic nervous system. We want that system happy, in pleasure, and full of power because it allows you to feel, well, Mojolicious!

The powers that be (God, Goddess, the Universe) are extraordinarily intelligent in the design of these human bodies. In the embryo stage, the cells that form the larynx are the same ones that form the ovaries. *And* when you look at a biological diagram of the throat and the vulva, they are nearly identical! I show a slide of each one at many of my live talks. I flip back and forth asking the audience which is which. They are literally aghast. Many whoas! and OMGs ripple through the audience. They don't teach us this in school (*shocker*, she says dripping with sarcasm). We must get this information out to as many women as possible. Because here's the deal, when you open your Self Expression Center, your Creative Center opens as well. And vice versa. When this happens, the world will be filled with women who are sexually empowered, self-expressed, and living life full of Mojo. No wonder the world is afraid to give us autonomy over our bodies. When we have it, we are unstoppable.

Back to activating your Self Expression Center.
It's time for Deep Throating.

Stay with me. You probably read that and thought, I'm out. I don't blame you if that was your initial reaction. Just the phrase brings up loads of misogynistic porn references with the focus on what the partner with the penis is getting out of it. Please hang in here and hear me out. Deep throating is a practice *for* you. You are about to learn the solo practice version. The main reason is so that you, *you m'dear*, can and will say what you want, when you want and how you want in and out of the bedroom. This is all about claiming your voice!

OK. Let's get your throat alive and moaning with pussy power!

Spirit Tools:

The following items can balance and invigorate the Self Expression Center. Use them prior to your practice to set the tone. You increase your spiritual sexual connection by combining these spirit tools with the sex ones.

◌ Anointing with Essential oils

This is the practice of smearing or rubbing your body with a substance to bless and consecrate your body as a sacred, energetic space. It connects the physical with the spiritual. It's most typically done with essential oils.

> **REMEMBER:** Use a carrier oil if you have sensitive skin. Almond, coconut, jojoba, olive oils are all good choices. You use a few drops of the essential oil with the carrier oil to make it easier on your skin and still reap the benefits.

Self-Expression Center: Dot the front of your throat *and* back of your neck. Your Self Expression Center, like all the others, goes from the front of your body to the back. Let's activate and anoint it powerfully.

Oils to use*:
* Sage (harmonious expression)
* Eucalyptus (clear, creative communication)
* Geranium (acceptance, confidence, stabilizing)
* Lavender (calming, relaxing)

◈ Elevating the Vibration with Crystals

* Using crystals (forms of minerals from the earth) is as ancient of a practice as soaking in mud baths to exfoliate and soften the skin. Have the crystals in the room where you choose to practice, sitting next to you or placed on your body.

Crystals to use*:

- Turquoise (expression, protection, spirit + earth integration)
- Sodalite (truth, verbalization of feelings, self-trust)
- Aquamarine (visioning, healing, self-love, freedom)
- Chalcedony (creative self-expression, calming, inner inspiration)
- Blue Lace Agate (articulate communication, purification)

♪ Create the Mood with Music*

When that certain song tickles your ears, your whole body gets excited. It's as if your inner dancer bursts out of your soul bathed in sequins, tassels, and go-go boots. She's giddy with life and the right music can do this for you too. Choose consciously.

Music to play:

- Any kind of music that's dominant with vocals. Ideally rich in high tones, meditative dance, or singing, or any New Age music. Think about the type of chanting that requires deep (pun intended) concentration and ability to regulate breathing. This can subconsciously support the awakening of your Self Expression Center.

👄 Sex Tools*:

The following items are where it's at to get your Self Expression Center humming and purring through Deep Throat play. I recommend working with the preparation practices first. A few days or a week will do the trick. Then move into the full practice. We want you a full *fuck yes* when you engage with the practice.

Water

Yep. Basic elixir of life. Have it on hand to keep your mouth and throat moisturized.

Hand Towel

Any will do. This is helpful for clean-up and intermittent wiping. We will be dealing with quite a bit of saliva during this practice.

Mini Spatula

You might notice a theme with the sex tools mentioned in this book. There are quite a few that cross the border from kitchen to bedroom and back again. Your mini spatula is one of those. I do recommend you have your *special* mini spatula for sexual practice only. You could have a few if that turns you on. They come in every color of the rainbow, some with designs and even logos. Choose one that tickles your pleasure.

Mini Dildo

The operative word here is *mini*. Our kind of Deep Throat practice is for *you*. This is not performative. Therefore, choose a mini dildo or at least one that is on the slimmer side. It does need to be long enough to reach the back of your mouth into your throat (keep that in mind). Dildos do not vibrate and they come in a variety of materials and colors. Choose one that makes you smile.

✧ Permission:

Give it to yourself.
It's underrated and makes a world of difference.
I am giving you permission right now.
You are worthy of owning your erotic nature.
Now claim it for yourself.
Say it aloud: *I AM worthy of owning my erotic nature.*

By reading these words you are free to experiment and play with yourself, relish in your sexuality, and connect it to your spiritual self. You are giving yourself a gift by doing so, and therefore, you are gifting the world. When you flourish, everyone around you will as well.

SOLO PLAY:

MIND

Deep Throat. Yes. You will gag (pay attention to the prep work. It puts your gag reflex on the lowest volume possible). And it's OK to gag. Your Self Expression Center is begging you to get on board. She has many lifetimes worth of dialogue to share. She craves sharing truth—loudly. She wants to cocreate a gorgeous, erotically alive existence with you.

You might need to let go of the idea that:

- Deep Throat is only the title of a well-known porn film
- only nasty, *bad girls* do such a thing
- this is only for people who do kinky, alternative sex things

- it's too scary to speak your truth
- women are better off silent
- vocalizing during sex is only for super confident women
- or any other idea you picked up

I realize the idea of Deep Throat practice can potentially be activating (I was *not* into it at first). What I know for sure is when you give yourself over to this practice, little miracles happen. They can be super subtle at first, like those faint rainbows. You're unsure if it's there but you see some colors penetrating the sky no matter how much you want to question it. As you open your Self Expression Center through your throat, you simultaneously expand your Creative Center. Don't blame me if you start to have exciting conversations and more pleasure on the daily. Get ready to claim your erotic nature.

Ready. Set. Open up and say ahhhhhhhh!

BODY

Let's take it slow.
Nice and easy.
This is about o-p-e-n-i-n-g.

Think of this part as preparing the table for a festive party. Sometimes the prep is fun because you're so excited about the event. Sometimes the prep feels more stressful because you want to get every little detail right. You might experience a combo of those feelings and then some. Welcome whatever comes to the surface. Similar to your cervix and the Creative Center, the throat has a significant history of withholds layered in it. This is the time to let that shit go. It could happen through tears, screams, laughter, a combination of those, or anything else. Please, m'dear, please do not hold back. This is the time for you to shed the years, and most likely generations, of restriction towards your communication. Remember, this erotic nature isn't exclusively about sex. Your erotic nature is about the way you BE. Your being-ness is the foundation for your overall experience of life. It's about the way you speak, eat, play, work, connect, create, and interact.

Make sure to stay hydrated. This helps with natural lubrication (both oral and vaginal). This practice can and most likely will, create an excess of saliva. In Level II, it will be a thicker saliva and that is excellent to assist with the practice.

Level I*

We begin the Deep Throat practice with addressing the gag reflex. Yep. Everyone's got it. It's a helpful function in general (don't want to get a piece of avocado toast lodged in there). Similar to the cervix and anus, the throat holds a lot of tension. Are you clenching your jaw as you read this? Yeah? That pulls on the muscles connected to the throat and neck, which layers in tension and restriction.

Claim this practice as sacred time with one, some, or all of these suggested intentions:

Say them aloud with as much Mojo as you can muster:

✧ It is safe to explore my erotic nature
✧ Being erotically alive feels good
✧ It's good to be erotically alive
✧ I love speaking my Truth
✧ Speaking my Truth is a contribution wherever I go

✧ I am empowered when I use my voice
✧ My voice is loving and powerful
✧ I express myself with ease and grace
✧ I love making all kinds of sounds with my voice

Take three deep breaths.
Inhale, yes. Exhale, release.
Inhale, pleasure. Exhale, tension.
Inhale, playfulness. Exhale, restriction.

Get yourself in a comfortable seated position with your mini spatula, water, and hand towel nearby. Begin by taking your mini spatula and slowly glide it on your tongue towards the back of your mouth. Remember to breathe. As soon as you feel the sensation of gagging arise, *pause*. Hold the spatula in your mouth and breathe deeply as you count backwards from ten. Then you can pull the spatula out completely.

Repeat this process nine times.

Each round see if you can take the spatula a little further back before the gag instinct kicks in. Always pause when it does, hold the spatula in your mouth and count backwards from ten. See how much relaxation you can experience during the countdown. Can you let your shoulders drop? Can you release the kung fu grip in your jaw? Are you able to sense energy in your cervix?

This process supports you in desensitizing your gag reflex. And look—do not feel bad if yours is holding on for dear life. It is built in to keep you alive AND most likely, it's been building strength over the years. Particularly if you are someone who's held your tongue more often than not.

Bonus Level I practice

It's helpful to practice desensitizing the gag reflex when you brush your teeth. So simple. So easy. Use your toothbrush similarly to the spatula except you brush your tongue. See how far back you can brush before the gag kicks in. As soon as you get the gah, gah *gag* feeling, pause with the toothbrush on your tongue, breathe and count backwards from ten.

Level II

It's time to soften, open and activate your Self Expression Center. There are three optimum positions for this level of the practice:

- Sitting on your knees (add a cushion between your legs if you have sensitive knees like me. This props you up a bit and takes the pressure off the knee joint).
- Straddling a small chair with your body facing the back of the chair so that your chest can press into it.
- Laying on your back on the bed with your neck hanging off the mattress.

Each of these positions assists in opening of the throat making for a more pleasurable and potent Deep Throat practice. Plus, they offer you ideal access to your sweet pussy because at some point you're going to want to do a combo platter practice of Self Expression Center and Creative Center. Kah-bam! Have fun and experiment with the positions to discover which one brings you most alive.

In your chosen position, take a few deep breaths. Let your body soften and relax. Use your dildo and gently begin inserting it in your mouth as far back as you can go. At this point, you are familiar with relaxing the gag reflex. If it arises, pause, hold the dildo in your mouth and count from ten to one. Pull it out and start again.

Experiment with exhaling fully as you take the dildo deeper into your mouth. When it reaches your throat, you will feel a "wall." Pause and hold the dildo there as you continue to breathe. Saliva may drip from your mouth—let it. *Be willing to get messy.* You will sense when it's time to pull the dildo out. Usually a few seconds is all it takes. Then take a moment, catch your breath, and go back into the practice. Allow a rhythm to emerge. Each time you take the dildo in see if you are able to hold it at the back of your throat for a moment longer than before. Eventually, your throat will yield to the dildo and it will move past the gag reflex and into the larynx. This new sensation might alarm you at first. It doesn't quite feel like anything else. The potential of pleasure is there for you, as awkward or bizarre as it might seem.

An additional trick to help you open the Self Expression center with the deep throating practice is humming. Yep. A little mmmm, mmmm, mmm, mm! You might have a tune that makes you feel like a Rockstar on stage. If you do, hum that one. Hum the tune that makes you feel the most empowered giving strength to your voice. The process of the hum lifts your soft palate (hello reducing gag reflex) and activates the vagus nerve. Win-win! I recommend adding in the hum when you are about to take the dildo into your throat. Let it be the segue between the moment of the pause and the actual deep throat.

Play with this technique for ten to fifteen minutes. It's a good amount of time to acclimate, open and activate the Self Expression Center. And be sure to always complete the practice on a *non-gag* run of the dildo. This helps to retrain your neural pathways and adopt the new erotically alive you as truth (vs. stopping the practice on a gag moment, which reinforces the old pattern and clamping down on your Self Expression Center).

SPIRIT*:

Get into a comfortable seated position in a quiet space where you can be undisturbed for five to fifteen minutes.

Light a candle if that inspires or feels good to you. A blue one symbolizes the Self Expression Center. In addition to the candle, incorporate any of the additional spirit tools you are drawn to use for this meditation.

Begin by taking three deep breaths.

Feel your consciousness sinking into your body.

Let whatever came before this moment go with each exhale as you sigh out an audible *ahhhhhh*.

Imagine the most loving, gentle, and nurturing energy appears in front of you. This energy can take the form of a being—it can be a human form, it can be an angelic or fairy form, it can be an amorphous form. However this energy emerges for you, allow it to bless you with its presence.

Take a deep breath.

This energy begins to glow as a clear, brilliant aquamarine light. The light waves dance in front of you like wisps of fabric blowing in the wind. In a moment, this clear, brilliant aquamarine light narrows down and transforms to a deeply condensed ball. The being moves the clear, brilliant aquamarine ball and gently places it on your throat. Like a queen receiving her royal jewel necklace, you sit a bit straighter and your shoulders drop down your back a smidge more.

The clear, brilliant aquamarine light feels warm against your skin. It's relaxing. You feel safe. The presence of the being diffuses into the space around you so that you are surrounded by this loving, accepting sensation from every direction.

In a moment, you will activate your Self Expression Center by making the sound of V. It will sound like *VUH* without the *UH*. It will be an elongated sound of V as you exhale. You do this by placing your lips together as you make the V sound on an exhale. You repeat this on every exhale for the duration of the practice. You start by repeating it for nine rounds and overtime, you work your way up to fifteen minutes of the practice without counting rounds.

To begin, feel the clear, brilliant aquamarine light around your neck.

Inhale the light.

Exhale with the V sound.

Allow the vibration to resonate in your Self Expression Center and beyond.

This is round one.

You continue the practice by repeating this breath and sound pattern.

Continue to complete nine full rounds.

Inhale the light.

Exhale with the V sound.

Allow the vibration to resonate in your Self Expression Center and beyond.

Return to your natural breath when you are complete.

Notice the sensation in your throat and back of the neck.

What is present for you now?

What, if anything, shifted in your body, mind and spirit?

This can be incredibly subtle. Be gentle with yourself. Just as the light-being offered you tender loving care, give that to yourself now.

When you are ready, open your eyes.

Welcome back.

* *Visit www.undressedbook.com for your free downloadable resource lists and guided meditation*

THIRD EYE

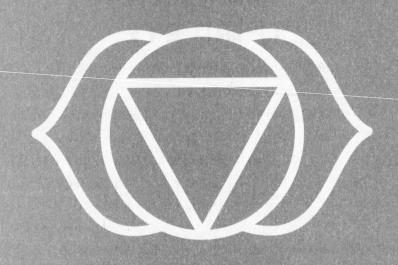

Power Center No. 6

WISDOM

Color: **INDIGO**

Sense: **EXTRASENSORY PERCEPTION**

Element: **N/A**

Physical Location: **FOREHEAD**

{the area just above the center of the brows}

Objective

The Wisdom Center is where you create tangible results from sheer thought. It is the place where you create the energy for the fulfillment of your desires. This center offers you insights past the physical and connects you with the knowledge of the unseen. Here is where you sharpen your intuitive abilities and communication with Spirit. Memory and concentration are natives of this center as well.

Harmony

With a fully functioning Wisdom Center, you perceive the world in its multi-dimensionality. The material world becomes transparent and you are able to decipher it for what it is—a dance of energy. Your purpose in the world is clear and following intuitive nudges is second nature. Seeing the bigger picture offers you healthy objective for your life. As well as the ability to be honest, loyal, and open minded.

Disharmony

You tend to be over analytical and too reliant on your intellect. Only the tangible aspect of life interests you. You deem spiritual insight or topics as unrealistic. Being stubborn and closed minded are your baselines. You tend towards confusion and mental stress. And you find personal growth, spiritual reflection, and visioning to be a waste of time.

Vivrant Thing

My mind is in overdrive. Every morning I barely get my eyes cracked and it's racing with thousands of obsessive thoughts. Apartment hunting, dating, emails, sex, exercise, state of the world, the skin on my thighs. My push-pull with life. It's totally exhausting. But noticing it all wows me. Not the "oh gee, isn't this terrific" kind of wow. The kind where I know I need to quiet it. This mind, which wants to steamroll the world of me, is exhausting. Amidst the ramblings this morning I realize, much to my surprise, I am still uncomfortable with intimate sex.

It's been easy to believe that I'm totally cool with sex. I know how much it fills me to be physical with another. The notion that being physical equates to being loved is something I've walked around with since my preteen years. It's deeper than simply being loved. It's about being of value in the world. Being sexual means I have purpose. That I'm necessary. That I'm cool because I'm the woman who can play like the boys. So, what's this other voice creeping into consciousness? The one saying it wants to be cherished? To be claimed. To be fucked into God? That mystical sensation of merging into everything holy. Where's that coming from? What does it mean?

For months I've read books about spiritual sex, getting to deeper levels of intimacy through sex, opening to higher levels of consciousness through sex. It's steeping in me. I want it. The old crusty layers of conditioning are splintering and it hurts. I know how well I've muffled the deep spiritual message center in my brain. This wound of love cuts so deep it feels as though my heart is pulverized, pouring forth its guts unabashedly. No barriers. No boundaries. Oozing love. That's all there is. Weaving its way through the energy.

Every Saturday for the last few months I haul my butt to an ashram an hour and a half away (with no traffic). This started because I was initiated into a spiritual practice called "shaktipat meditation." The kick off happened at a six-day silent meditation retreat. Yeah. Absolutely no talking whatsoever for six whole days with thirty-four other people doing the same. We ate meals together. Did yoga together. Slept in yurts together. Swam in the creek together. We never said a word to each other. I found it oddly comforting. I didn't need to stay so attached to my personality. I wasn't worried about being clever, funny, smart, or even remotely noticed. Blending into the spaces between the silence became a pleasure. I wondered why we ever needed to talk again because so much is communicated with a glance or body movement. And it's much easier to appreciate everyone else when they don't say anything. OK. There's still judgment going on from the visuals (why is that woman wearing short shorts when her legs are barely long enough to carry her? He thinks he's so cool doing bakasana like it's a no brainer. If they eat all those beans it's going to be a stinky night). But when they don't open their mouths to speak—wow! The thick distinctive lines separating them from me become light. Almost fuzzy. By day six the idea that we're all one is much closer to truth than ever before.

The shaktipat meditation hooks me. Three of the five nights at the retreat our group sits faithfully in the yoga room lit by candles. A recording of a Sanskrit mantra (sacred prayer) sounds over and over on the stereo as the group chants along with it. This is the only time we are allowed to use our voices. The teacher, a long-time devout yogi dresses in loose flowing Indian pants, tunic top adorned with metallic embroidery, and sandalwood paste smeared on his forehead, walks around holding a cluster of peacock feathers. Kind of like the spiritual version of a cat o' nine tails. He stands behind each person, mutters something, and then starts whacking their back with the feathers. The droning of the group chanting swells at times, making it all feel a little cultish. Some people have major "releasing" upon their shaktipat. People will moan or make animal noises or scream or cry. Bodies shake like earthquakes or fall to the ground. It is said that these are "normal" reactions to shaktipat since the experience is meant to awaken your kundalini—*the* Life Force living inside you. When awakened, it can catapult through you and dissolve emotional, spiritual, psychological, or physical blockages, which show up in a variety of bizarre ways. If I wasn't so dedicated to connecting to my/the Higher Source, I would've gone running for the highway to hitch a ride back to the good ol' world of numb materialism. But those thick lines that normally keep us separated from one another are no longer there. The energy in the room rapidly transforms into an ocean of smoke. We are wisps mingling. You can't tell who is who. We all simply are.

I think I might vomit when it comes time for me to get whacked. A surge of fear races through me. I remember to tell myself to focus on breathing. My mind argues, wanting me to chant and stay with the group. *Whack.* Feathers on my lower back. *Ho!* Energy splatters open at the base of my spine. *Whack.*

Feathers on my lower back. Explosion. *Whack*. Feathers on my lower back. Fireworks. *Whack Whack*. Feathers move up my spine. Technicolor lava shoots up my back. *Whack*. Body begins uncontrollable shaking. *Whack Whack Whack*. Unearthly sound erupts from my mouth. *Whack*. What the fuck is happening? *Roll with it*. Who's that? *Get into it*. Wha...? *Let go*. It's like having a whole-body orgasm and my body is pure light. At that moment, the teacher puts his thumb on my third eye while he gently brushes my back in upward strokes with the feathers. Total mind-numbing calm penetrates my body as my neck spontaneously whips back and my entire spine becomes crescent moon shaped. Mouth fully open, breath inhaling like Darth Vader's spiritual twin—I am frozen. I have no idea what is happening. I am into it. A sweet tap on the top of the head with the feathers and I snap back into the room.

My life will never be the same. I am smitten to the point that I make the trek every weekend for three months to bask in the bliss that is shaktipat meditation. I feel closer to Truth than ever before. I feel oddly intimate with myself. Like I have a secret handshake with my soul. And it's good. Until I start to see a clique forming amongst some of the followers. This sets off an alarm in my personal psychic security system. I observe. It is when the "guru" blows into my mouth during shaktipat that I know there is something amiss here. There is something sexual about it and it feels entirely out of place during what is supposed to be a sacred practice. Those two things are still separated in my consciousness. And, I don't see him do this blowing in mouth bit with any of the men. Plus, I'm hiding my true desire of reaching that place, the one where spirit and sex meet, with a man. I continue to long for a divine sexual connection. A merging of energies between bodies, all while worshipping one another in the act of loving sex. This whole part about finding God through sex totally interests me and I am not clear on how to proceed.

Careful what you ask for—cuz here he is. We see each other whenever he passes through town. As usual, he looks like a wandering prophet walking along the side of the road. He is literally a man about the world. Wherever he goes, there he is, and he belongs to no one and nowhere. I find this fascinating and odd. It's something I envy and despise, which keeps me coming back for more with him. My car pulls up and he sidles over to the driver's side window. His long 6'4" frame curves down to greet my face. Chest-length gray hair is pulled into a loose ponytail. His usual adornments, oversized mala beads and a leather wrapped long jade carving from his native land of New Zealand, peek out from his half buttoned pink shirt. He smells travel weary, musty with a crisp smack of cool. His face is inches from mine.

"Well hello there. Need a ride?" I say in my best breathy Marilyn Monroe.

He laughs, long fingered hands holding his belly and something about the way he tosses his head back reminds me of a cackling crone—it's surprisingly sexy. I realize he's one of the few men I know that effortlessly embodies and blends the feminine with masculine. It gives him a sense of sweet coating his rough edges— the modern Frappuccino.

He leans down again, this time to kiss my lips. He takes a taste. Pauses. And comes back for some more. His tongue reaches for mine through his parted lips. It's welcomed in my hungry mouth. The sound of a car horn blasts from behind my car and startles us back to reality. "Get in," I say through my giggles. He circles the car and slides into the passenger side. We sit there, frozen in each other's gaze. He blinks slowly and with purpose. This is his way of connecting to me. Of letting me know he is *here*, present, and acknowledging all that we are in the moment. I soak it in. Him, us, the seeming insanity of it all, and the perfection. Another horn blasting whips me back and I put the car in gear ready to drive back to my apartment. It's always at my place because he has no home. We only see each other every six weeks or so, and when we are together it is for a mere handful of hours.

I'm a bit shocked that he connects to what I put out. I remember lying in my bed a few months ago reading his recently published book on intimacy and sacred sexuality. I thought, "It would be amazing to have him be the one to work on sex/love/God/connecting." Whallah! It happened.

The first time he comes over, I prepare a smattering of food. Very Mediterranean—hummus, olives, good bread, lovely salad, and my favorite cheese, La Tur. The table is set for a "special" guest and I wonder why I am making the fuss. I can hear my grandmother whispering in my ear, *every guest in your home should feel special*. At that moment, I know I am kidding myself. I want to seduce this man, not knock him over the head with it. No. Titillate his senses to the point where he wants me to be the next dish. I am giddy like a schoolgirl waiting for him. When he stands in my doorway that first time, I wonder if he is just an occasion for me to see myself? Feel myself? They talked of "occasions" in the shaktipat ashram. These are people who appear in one's life to foster a lesson or experience. It's all under the guise of inner growth—if you can stay detached enough from it and realize it's only "an occasion" and not something to believe as absolute truth. As he sits across the Indian teak dining room table from me, I know. It's all good. Moment to moment. We'll see. No expectations

The second time, he stands in my doorway feigning rock 'n roll cool—arm up against the doorjamb, slouchy posture, one knee bent.

"Hey babe," he says in his best American accent covering the native Kiwi.

"Hey yourself."

He shoves a CD in my face.

"This is you. 'The Goddess in the Doorway'."

I look at the same-titled Rolling Stones CD in his hand.

"Well. Come on in and let's put it on."

Continuing his cool routine, he swaggers in laughing. He glances at me with clear blue eyes that can look so feminine and fill with mischief when I make him laugh. I feel at the mercy of my open wanting heart around him.

He takes me in his arms and dips me halfway to kiss me with his thin lips. All of this melts me. His smell is musty with BO and yet sweet on his skin. The road worn hands embracing my body are a total turn on. He spots the tea and fig cookies on the table. I know they are his favorite and I make a point of having them on hand when he visits. I want him to have me first. But there's a ritual to this dance. I follow the steps dutifully because the payoff is big, however amorphous.

We sit on the living room floor, spines erect, facing one another. He tilts his head down and his eyes up—penetrating into mine. Blink. Slight nod and blink. It's his "energy hook up." A swift motion of his hand commands me to sit astride him. I do as asked. I am nervous and eager. Up to this point, we have only shared kisses and light touching. This is a new moment. A new level. I carefully place myself over him, legs wrapping his waist. My nearly foot shorter frame settles easily into his lap. He stays completely connected to me through his eyes and breath. It's as if he is breathing me. My inhales begin to match his and then my exhales. That separating line, the one that our bodies make, begins to blur and my insides heat up. The shaktipat meditation kind of heat. He pulls back for a moment. Can he sense the start of the surge welling in me? Maybe so because he pulls his t-shirt over his head and tosses it to the couch. Soft tan skin covers the length of him. His nipples are the kind I've always envied. They stand up and point at me, daring me to suckle and nibble on them. They are perfect protrusions from his chest; another sign he's both masculine and feminine in one body. He kisses me, soft and then deep.

"Yum," gurgles from his mouth.

"Mm," I moan.

His hand cradles the base of my spine. Oh, there is that heat. He presses harder. Oh boy. Harder still. *Whoosh.* I am taken by the surges of pure life force soaring through my body. He sends the shakti up through me and holds the space for all of it. My body shakes like it did at the retreat. It feels as if I'll lose control and fall apart in pieces. It is scary and invigorating. I feel him all through my body. At least I think that is him. And what is that? A flash of deep sadness wells up, tinged with fear. The fear feels linked to the sexual shame that still lives within me. Before I can tightly wrap my mind around it, it's gone. Like the ocean settling to the shore, I smooth out. It is the most intense complete orgasmic experience without having intercourse, without even taking my clothes off. Who knew? He leans his forehead against mine. The weight of our knowledge co-mingling creates a larger-than-life feeling in me. My body is swollen and I am nine feet tall. All those years of seeking profound experiences through sex and now the sex isn't even a factor to get there. Wild. I feel grateful he showed up in my life. The combination of his wisdom and my openness makes a tight fit. I like it.

The weeks between seeing him aren't painful. I find this somewhat startling because the me I'm used to would be pining away, waiting for the next moment he'd walk in my door, wondering when he'd want to fuck me. Or why hadn't he fucked me. Instead, I deal with the day to day. A new reality emerges. One where I can be excited about seeing him without getting crushed. One where I know the sex isn't the main attraction. He touches base with me about once a week. A phone call. An email. As far off and free as he might be, he keeps the energy connection alive between us. The fact that I literally manifested him into my life still tickles me. Yes, I showed up at a class he was teaching to initially connect with him. But that was only to hear him speak about his work and newly released book. I never thought my idea of him as a lover could become real. Now that it is, I have conviction in my ability to create life. The fact that I can tune into THE consciousness, focus on a desire with strong feeling, and watch it materialize is a blast.

He calls on my birthday and sings me a chant. I'm not sure where he was calling from and I don't care. Hearing his voice expands my heart, lifts my spirit. He continues his chant and I literally feel him moving in me. Whatever energy/life-force he triggers makes its way round my body. The space just above my eyebrows in the center starts to hum. He ends the chant with my name. He repeats it over and over as if it is a sacred mantra. I think this is funny at first. Hearing it repeated more than twice, I settle in like a chided schoolgirl, recognizing there is something special going on.

"Why don't you go to the Vedanta Temple in Hollywood."

I previously shared my weird experience with a picture of a saint during all those months of shaktipat meditation. Basically, one night after the whole peacock feather-whacking shindig, I wanted to look at all the photos of the saints in the room. There were a dozen or so three by four foot framed photos lining the walls. Looking at each of them, into their eyes, I wondered what made them so special. Or any different than me. And when I stood in front of the saint named Ramakrishna, an energy whip cracked my spine and I instantly fell into a bout of the uncontrollable shakes. To say this was weird is an understatement. To tell the next part still embarrasses me. There I was having these kriyas (that's what they call this kind of release) and I was looking right at Rama's face as it started to morph into another face. One that looked vaguely like all the images of the Buddha—shaved head, round cheeks, happy smile. As soon as I thought "wow", it started to morph into another face and then another until this cacophony of faces fuzzed out leaving no face whatsoever. The neck was there. But no face. A blank void.

I have never taken hallucinogens, nor have I ever wanted to. But, this felt like the closest experience to them without actually doing them. Either that or the shaktipat thing was actually a cult and someone put something real funky in the rice pudding. But wait. I didn't eat the pudding until after the experience. The whole thing knocked the wind out of me.

"Will you go to the Vedanta temple?" he inquires again.

"Uh, OK. Where is it?"

"Off Gower and the 101. There's a lot of Ramakrishna inside. I think it'd be good for you." Even from out of town he likes to educate me. Nice. He is like an ambassador. His energy is like that. Someone who opens up doorways for people to expand, understand life (and themselves) better.

I pause, considering it before replying, "OK. My girlfriend is taking me out to dinner. But I can swing by before I meet her."

"Good."

Sex is overrated. Sex in general. These thoughts yank my mind's eye as I sit in the incense-filled space. The temple, resting on the hill above a hectic commuter highway, is the calm to the urban storm. The Shakti to the Shiva outside. As much as I thought I liked consummating the physical urge of animal gratification when my loins get stirred, it becomes crystal clear—if my soul isn't in the building, it's a nonstarter. That's where I feel empty. The voice of one of my sex and intimacy teachers whispers through my consciousness. *Have sex as a gift. Receive sex as a gift. Be full of Love desire—then have sex.* I take a deep breath thinking, *"Exactly! Truly connected and spiritually inspired sex is divine."*

We end up on my bed. This is a first. An upgrade from the living room. Our clothes are off, save for the underwear—very matter of fact. No sexplay with the disrobing process. I admire his long, lean, and tanned body. The sparkle in his blue eyes grows purposeful and I am almost intimidated by his presence. I want him physically. I can already feel him. My fear is the thing in the room that I can't identify. It is the feeling that something besides the sex is happening. Like at the ashram in front of the picture of Ramakrishna. I know I was there and there was no control. Part of me is grasping for the known—have sex, be in the physical act, attach to it. The other part is clamoring at my psychospiritual walls, making its great escape into the next realm. The one where polarities merge. The one of utter surrender to another. The one of healing through intimate connection.

He remains focused. Steady. As he lays me down on the bed I feel myself soften, giving over to this moment. He has me on my back with his left arm behind my shoulders, holding me close. He is on his side leaning over me. His kiss is the breath of life. The oxygen between us is liquid. Our mouths melt as tongues lap at our combined elixir.

He takes my hand, tucks it in his underwear and places it on his greatness, "I want you to feel what you're dealing with."

Electric waves crash through my body and I flail in ecstasy. How can this simple hand to skin connection create such intense pleasure? I feel his hard-on and it is a force to be reckoned with. The depth of his presence swells in his loins, as I grow hungry for him. I suddenly need him in my mouth. I take him as though I am worshipping at the temple of every man. His cock is glorious. Large thick head with an equally magnificent shaft. It quakes me to look at it. He won't let me capture all of him. He is not anticipating my desire to taste him. He pulls me back.

Again, on the left side of him with his left arm wrapped behind my shoulder, he takes his right hand down to my sex. He cups my underwear-clad mound and holds me. Light streams up through me and I am taken. I'll do anything he wants. I feel more feminine than ever before. I let myself completely surrender to him in that moment. He pushes my panties down my legs and I wiggle them off my feet. He explores the flesh of my sex. His thick fingers take in the velvet essence as a throaty *"mmm"* sounds through the bedroom. Is that him or me? Now his fingers plunge in. *Whack.* It is like the peacock feathers are stroking me from the inside out. Body shudders. *Whack Whack.* Fingers so deep inside it is as if he is going to rip my heart out through my pussy. The old me wants to clamp down. Stay rigid. Stick to the known. The larger part of me, the truth of me, wants to unfurl. To blast open and witness the claiming. *Whack.* The energy running through my spine is intense. I succumb to the joy and pain, all together.

"Yum," he says kissing me. "Yum…" as though he is tasting nectar.

"Hold my breasts," he commands. Taking his hand out of me, he takes my hand and places it on his chest.

I can't see straight and I am losing touch with whose body is whose. It doesn't matter. I am swimming in the sea of this bliss. Finding his chest, I grab his nipples, pinch, and pull them as he moans, "Yes, yes." And "Thank you." His always erect nipples are gorgeous. I love sucking them. They remind me of a woman's breasts. And I realize that, though he is a man, very much so, there's an androgynous energy about him. He encapsulates such a wellspring of knowledge in the esoteric realm that it is as if he can shapeshift. I am totally turned on. Like having the best of both worlds in one being.

Without moving much, he slides on top of me and looks me straight in the eyes. Then purposefully blinks. Yes. I am here. I am actually petrified, but I am there. It is confirmed in real time now— even if my loins are stirred, I can feel the disconnect from my soul. And that is where I felt empty. With him, laying over me, about to enter me, I feel hyper connected. Like suddenly being thrust into college, straight out of kindergarten. He continues to gaze into my eyes while his hand finds his cock. Strong and slow—he enters me. *Whack*. A mantra whispers on his lips. He is actually chanting something. I do all I can to stay in one piece. Rocket fuel races up and down my spine. My breath is deep. At the bottom of an exhale there is a swarm of butterflies tickling my uterus. *Pump. Thrust.*

"Thank you."

Hearing him utter these words seems strange. Why is he thanking me? *Whack*. Oh. Amidst this frenzy, a lightning bolt of revelation punctures my awareness. He is not thanking *me*—he is thanking The Energy. The Mother. The Feminine. The Force that he is accessing through us. It is this moment that I become consciously aware of the connection to all things. That we are the full-blown intelligence of life. His body, his personality is an occasion for me to feel that depth of knowledge and collective consciousness, eternally available.

"Can you take more?" he looks into my eyes and beyond them.

"Yes. Oh yes." I moan.

Thrust. Thrust. His upper body barely moves as his pelvis continues to rock my world. One hand is tucked under me at the base of my spine, the other right behind my neck, cradling my skull. *Whack.* Here come the shudders. Body quaking, earth shaking shaktipat meditation gyrating. I can't see straight. I don't care.

"Oh, you take it so good. Oh yes," he says in a half chant, half growl.

The fact that this man chants mantras *and* talks a little dirty to me makes me come unglued. It's polarities merging. It's opposites in one place. The sacred and profane. It is exactly what I've been craving. The stark truth, staring me in the shrunken fullness of my being, cracks me open. *Yes! This is me.* I take in air through my nostrils, warm and dense, while his cock fills me below. I unfurl from both ends and let life into my body. Skin and bones and walls and furniture and everything tangible evaporates. I am unaware of any separation. Now all I feel is one breathing pulsing gushing oozing life force swirling everywhere. I access Truth here. Love is all there is here. The dramas of—does he like me? What am I doing with my life? Am I pretty? Is the world falling apart? How can we survive like this?—vanish. There is nothing more relevant than this.

He chants a seed mantra. It's one word in a low humming tone. He repeats this over and over. The vibration radiates my entire being. I can feel the rush of familiar sexual build up happening in my pussy. I almost don't want to cum. It seems silly. Slightly crass in the context of all this beauty. But he pumps me knowingly, coaxing me to climax. I give in to the moment. Utterly surrendering to him as he does to me. All the rocket fuel that pooled in my groin lights up. It burns bright and explodes up my belly and spine. When it reaches the center of my chest I feel like I can't breathe. It gets to my throat. I gasp for air, pulling it down the front of my body. His fingertips press into the base of my skull, acting as an anchor. Peacock feathers are everywhere. The skin I once knew vibrates at such a high speed I can't feel it. It is as if I am completely swollen. I am inside myself, yet bigger. And then, it comes. The flood of tears. Climax and crying. I am wide open, feeling so much that tears stream silently out of me. My mind tries to clamor on and be embarrassed. It doesn't matter. My mind is weak in that moment. His knowing hand lovingly strokes the center of my forehead.

"Ah yes. The blissful body wet with tears."

I manage a smile.

"Beautiful," he kisses my mouth.

I wake up the next morning, not exactly sure what happened. He is up doing his morning yoga practice in the living room. I quietly stand in the doorway watching him. He is stunning. Grace in motion. As the sunlight peeks in the window, I see it. I see the light of the masculine and feminine interacting as him—his physical being that of the masculine and his devotion fully of the feminine. I see the merging of the polarities in him. I see the window opening to profound layers of life. I feel my own pleasure and the wide, freshly paved pathways in my body. I can see things in a way I haven't yet seen them. I feel more claimed by life than ever before.

YOUR TURN

Wisdom Center

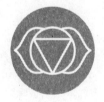

The connection to our higher self, intuition, and divine knowings are all connected here. This center is known as the "spiritual voice and message center." Sometimes it's referred to as the Truth portal. Clarity, development of the inner senses, mind power, projection of the will, and manifestation are key aspects.

Wanna know why your intuition is often referred to as your sixth sense?

I think it is directly related to the fact that your sixth energy center is your third eye. The seat of knowing beyond the physical facts. The space where you connect with the wisdom of the universe on a vibrational level. The sixth energy center *is* the gateway to receiving intuitive pings. Coincidence?! Maybe. I don't have hard data to back this up *and* you can find endless correlations to the invisible realms of life that are frankly too close to ignore. This seems to be one of them.

Women's intuition is to be revered. Sadly, you and I both know that has *not* been the case for way too long. It's been called crazy, silly, ridiculous, nonsense—and the one that gets my pussy inflamed (not in a good way!), hysterical. The barrage of insults, gaslighting, and defamation of women's intuition is horrendous. The collective denigration towards women's intuition bleeds into your personal experience, acceptance, and confidence with it.

Having unshakable capacity with your Wisdom Center is critical to owning your erotic nature. It allows you to tap into your higher wisdom, open up to your Truth, and create your desires in a tangible, earthly form.

To activate your Wisdom Center, we're going triple X.

Porn baby, PORN!

Get ready to elevate your fantasies. This is where you connect them with your sex *and* spirit. Through choosing higher vibration media, your capacity with the Wisdom Center skyrockets.

Now, like all things in this book, we're not going for the patriarchal version of this tool. We are looking at it through an empowered lens. One where women are *the* consideration. One where women are *the* creators. One that allows you to see a woman's pleasure is *the* portal to receiving and accepting more of your own.

The idea of porn can be confronting. Many people do not consider it erotic. When, in fact, the erotic is inherently connected to porn.

Merriam-Webster's definition of pornography is:

1. the depiction of erotic behavior (as in pictures or writing) intended to cause sexual excitement
2. material (such as books or a photograph) that depicts erotic behavior and is intended to cause sexual excitement
3. the depiction of acts in a sensational manner so as to arouse a quick intense emotional reaction

When we look at porn through its definition, it can be less threatening. Think about it—something that causes sexual excitement. Don't you want that? Don't you want to be aroused and feel erotically alive?! Since you are here, reading this, my guess is: *you bet!*

Spirit Tools:

The following items can balance and invigorate the Wisdom Center. Use them prior to your practice to set the tone. You increase your spiritual sexual connection by combining these spirit tools with the sex ones.

◌ Anointing with Essential Oils

This is the practice of smearing or rubbing your body with a substance to bless and consecrate your body as a sacred, energetic space. It connects the physical with the spiritual. It's most typically done with essential oils.

Wisdom Center: Dot the space in the middle of your forehead just above your eyebrows. You can press your palm into this area when anointing. Imagine a gentle, *oh geez* forehead in palm moment. Just like all the other centers, this one goes from the front of the forehead to the back of the head. You can press your other palm into the back of the head when you anoint if that feels best.

Oils to use*:
* Mint (clears, brightens, stimulates)
* Jasmine (deepens truth, sharpens senses)
* Pine or Sandalwood (integrates spiritual energies)

◈ Elevating the Vibration with Crystals

Using crystals (forms of minerals from the earth) is as ancient and trendy of a practice as dying your hair with henna. Have the crystals

UNDRESSED

in the room where you choose to practice, sitting next to you or placed on your body.

Crystals to use*:
- Amethyst (trust, devotion, receptive)
- Fluorite (mental clarity + peace of mind)
- Azurite (enhances intuitive ability)
- Sapphire (purifying, transforming, renewing)

♪ Create the Mood with Music*

Choose music that makes your body ready to move, groove, and awaken. If you choose to play music during your practice, make sure it *opens* you up.

Music to play:
Sacred songs are recommended. Any kind that opens you to cosmic dimensions, new age, any style of classical. Bach is noted. If you follow a particular spiritual tradition that has hymns, chants, or instrumental music that enlivens you, you can listen to that as well.

👄 Sex Tools*:

The following are where it's at to get your Wisdom Center alive and kickin' through porn play. I recommend practicing and experimenting with them all, but not all at once. We don't want to hyper stimulate your Wisdom Center and blast it to outer space. Each tool provides a specific nuanced sensation, therefore helping you reach a new threshold in your capacity for power and pleasure.

Screen

If you've got a device and internet, you have access to porn. Here is where you can explore videos, movies, erotic, and titillating content. There are many resources these days to explore great adult content*. Content that can and will light you up. Be mindful though, not all porn sites are built alike. Many of them can contain computer viruses. Just like engaging in any sexual activity, use protection and be aware.

You might be an eBook reader, and if so, your screen is also a place to devour some delicious erotica in the form of stories.

Sound

Thanks to sex and sexuality becoming more and more accepted at large, we have great innovations like audio porn*. This is where you can listen to a wide range of voices, genders, and erotic encounters.

Page

For old school ladies like myself, the page is where it's at. A real live and in the flesh book. With pages. With a smell. With a specific shape and size. Reading erotica from an old-fashioned paper book can do wonders for you.

✧Permission:

Give it to yourself.
It's underrated and makes a world of difference.

I am giving you permission right now.

You are worthy of owning your erotic nature.

Now claim it for yourself.

Say it aloud: *I AM worthy of owning my erotic nature.*

By reading these words you are free to experiment and play with yourself, relish in your sexuality, and connect it to your spiritual self. You are giving yourself a gift by doing so, and therefore, you are gifting the world. When you flourish, everyone around you will as well.

SOLO PLAY:

MIND

Porn. Does the idea of it make you cringe? Or are you like, sister please! I love my porn and proud to say it. Maybe you're somewhere in the middle. Any way you slice this pie, there's stigma around the word, and certainly, the art form.

What we know for sure is that it's been around for thousands of years. Which is a great thing because it punctuates that humanity, from the get-go, has had sexual and erotic desires. So much so that they felt the need to document it. I mean, if it's not important, would they have taken all that time to carve it in the dark caves when they had to survive sabretooth tigers and shit?

The Kangjiashimenji Petroglyphs in Xinjiang, the north-west region of China, depict some kind of orgy. Brazil is home to what's known as "Little Horny Man"—the oldest erotic rock carving, dating back 11,000 years, and depicts a man with a cock nearly as big as his arm. Multiple temples in India are home to gorgeous erotic carvings, within and beyond their walls; all created in the second century.

The debate between what is erotic art and what is porn continues. I suspect it will for as long as we live because it feeds into the patriarchal systems of controlling women, shaming women for their erotic natures, and making women wrong for being sexually and sensually vibrant.

And, in order for you to fully awaken to your erotic nature, it's critical that you open the Wisdom Center.

You might need to let go of the idea that:

- porn is only for lonely, creepy men
- all porn degrades women
- women are victims in the porn industry
- watching porn makes you gross or unlovable
- there isn't any porn that turns you on
- or any other ideas you picked up

I realize it might seem absurd to you to integrate porn into your life. Particularly when you are awakening your Wisdom Center. But remember m'dear, your erotic energy, that life force *is* the creative juice of the Universe. Channel *that* energy with an extra smidge of pure sex energy and you've got some seriously potent manifestation Mojo. *And* when you combine all of that with your inner vision, well, you're unstoppable.

So, let's crack out the proverbial Windex® and wipe your Wisdom Portal spanking clean.

BODY

Bust out that Kindle!

Fire up your laptop!

Coax that book off the shelf!

It's time to open your pleasure portal through accessing new layers of eroticism with porn.

This is your time to play, experiment, go into the potential kinks and potent fantasies you've been curious about—yet, haven't let yourself play on that street.

This is the time to stretch yourself. No one needs to know... unless YOU want them to know.

Been curious about same gendered sex? Ménage à trois? Or Foursome? Or Orgy? What about bondage? What about vulva worship? Does the idea of erotic massage light you up?

There's *something* in the realm of the erotic that's made its way across the dance floor of your mind. Go check that out.

Once you pick your flavor and delivery medium, make sure you're in a safe, private spot.

Claim this practice as sacred time with one, some, or all of these suggested intentions. Say them aloud with as much Mojo as you can muster.

✦ It is safe to claim my erotic nature

✦ I am worthy of living with erotic energy every day

✦ It is my choice to explore my sex and sexuality how I please

✦ I love my deep, private erotic fantasies

✦ Exploring my fantasies through porn is a conscious and safe erotic expression

✦ Engaging with porn gives me permission to expand sexually

✦ I learn to appreciate my sexuality through conscious use of porn

✦ When I can see what I want, I can create it

✧ The more I honor my erotic vision, the more I accept myself

Before you hit play on your device or open the page…
Take three deep breaths.
Inhale, yes. Exhale, release.
Inhale, pleasure. Exhale, tension.
Inhale, playfulness. Exhale, restriction.

Let's make sure you are grounded *in* your body while you engage in the porn. The interesting thing about working with the higher energy centers is how easy it is to float up and away. True erotic nature is anchored in your body while simultaneously connected to higher wisdom.

Now, your scene is as important, if not more, than the one you're watching, listening to, or reading. Get yourself situated in a yummy, delish surrounding. How's the lighting? What are you wearing (or not wearing)? Do you have a preferred beverage near-by? Make yourself feel like a Goddess worshiping at her own temple.

As you get into the porn, challenge yourself to consciously breathe. You will find that you're probably holding your breath. It's normal. One good belly breath will bring you back to presence in your body and that helps to integrate and assimilate the porn. Let your body get hot. Let yourself get turned on. Let your pussy swell. And let your vision of what's possible peel wide open.

Stay focused. Stay present. You might want to tune out. Catch yourself. Take a deep belly breath. Continue on.

You can imagine yourself in the porn scene or scenario. It's also perfectly acceptable to imagine yourself in the scene or any other with someone you fantasize about—the person you reserve for the privacy of your own mind. Does that make you quiver with fear? Or flush you with a fiery hot *fuck yes*? Imagine what it would be like for you to have this fantasy or desire. Can you allow yourself to be that free?

In the early stages of this practice, I encourage you to stay with the porn only. Meaning, no self-pleasuring. Focus on what you're experiencing through the porn. Notice what's happening to your body. Where are your thoughts? And for sure, be vigilant with your breath practice. Let the breath be your guide and grounding stone (the suggested gemstones can also help you open the Wisdom Center while being in the body).

Once you develop a friendship with porn, *then* incorporate self-pleasure if you'd like. See how present you can stay with the scene, your body, and your vision. It's a lot to tackle and it's a potent way to claim your erotic nature.

SPIRIT*:

Sit in a quiet space where you can be undisturbed for five to fifteen minutes.

Light a candle if that inspires or feels good to you. An indigo one symbolizes the Wisdom Center. In addition to the candle, incorporate any of the additional spirit tools you are drawn to use for this meditation.

Begin by taking a few deep breaths.
Sink into your body.
Let whatever came before this moment float away like wisps of incense smoke.

Gently close your eyes.

Now, place the tip of your tongue on your upper palate.

The spot right after the upper ridged area just as the skin becomes smooth.

This point supports opening your Wisdom Center as you engage in the spirit practice.

Continue to breathe consciously through your nose.

Slow and steady.

Next, with your eyes still closed, look up to the point just above the bridge of your nose. This is another way to activate the Wisdom Center. Do your best to keep your eyes and tongue in these positions for the whole practice.

Now, visualize a small kaleidoscope wheel in your Wisdom Center—located between your eyebrows, slightly above the brow bone. The wheel pulses. It begins to move organically, revealing patterns of shapes, colors, and sizes. It feels magical and alive.

The kaleidoscope begins to slow down. The spinning transitions to a pulsing. A steady beat. The beat begins to take pace with your heartbeat. Thump. Thump thump. Thump. The kaleidoscope beat, now aligned with your heart, slowly turns an indigo color. It is a round, throbbing, indigo-colored brilliant light. As if the most precious amethyst stone is implanted in your Wisdom Center. The beat carries on, and with each pulse it begins to grow. The gem becomes fuller and wider. Like a sacred cone emanating from your third eye. It grows outward with each pulse until the stunning indigo light is bigger and wider than your entire body.

Take three deep breaths.
Inhale possibility. Exhale restriction.
Inhale pleasure. Exhale irritation.
Inhale enthusiasm. Exhale frustration.

Now, from this space of enlivened opening, ask a question. What's
something you desire deeper understanding about. Something that
might be weighing heavily on you. Something that could bring a
sense of inner freedom once you receive clarity.

The question could be about your sexuality.
The question could be about your connection to spirit.
The question could be about a specific situation.

You can start your inquiry by saying:
Please let me see...
And fill in your question from there.
What would truly open you up right now?
Allow that to bubble up to your Wisdom Center and place it in
this ethereal indigo light.
Take three deep breaths.
Notice what occurs.
Simply notice.
The wisdom may arrive in colors, words, feelings, or symbols.
Allow the information to arise.

If you become distracted, check the placement of your tongue.
Make sure the tip is on the soft palate and press it upwards
three times to re-engage the connection. Notice where your eyes
are focused. If they drifted from the upward gaze, refocus on the
area just above the bridge of your nose with your eyes still closed.

Breathe into your belly.
Feel the wisdom from your third eye sink low into your body.
Allow the connection to be bold. Potent. Clear.
Surrender to the information coming through you.

When you are complete with receiving the wisdom, imagine the shining indigo cone draws back towards your third eye. Once it is fully back, it again becomes a throbbing, glistening gemstone pulsing to your heartbeat. Imagine a small window or door opens in your wisdom center. The indigo gemstone easily floats into it and backwards about an inch into your forehead. The window or door gently closes.

Take three deep belly breaths.
Welcoming the storehouse of wisdom.
Owning the portal to your wisdom.
Trusting it is available anytime you desire.
When you feel complete, relax your tongue and slowly flutter your eyes open.
Welcome back.

* Visit www.undressedbook.com for your free downloadable resource lists and guided meditation

CROWN

Power Center No. 7

ONENESS

Color: **WHITE + GOLD**

Sense: **DIVINE CONNECTION**

Element: **N/A**

Physical Location: **TOP OF HEAD**

{the physical top of your head and the space above it}

Objective

The Oneness Center is the space that connects you to the All. This is where you experience connection to the Divine and a sense of completeness. A deeper understanding and discovery of universal mystery is available to you through this center. You connect heaven and Earth here. This is the place where you wake up.

Harmony

You love and understand people. There is an acceptance of the fact that you are a vessel for the Divine. You live a joyful life connected to your spiritual values. When hardships arise, you have the wherewithal to overcome them. There is a limitless quality to your self-expression. Living aligned with the concept of heaven on earth is your baseline.

Disharmony

You feel disconnected from universal abundance. A sense of separateness pervades your life. You lean towards skepticism and lack inspiration most days. Apathy and boredom are your baselines. There's a palpable sense of distrust in yourself, life, and others. Superficiality is your comfort zone. And extreme attachment to the physical world consumes you.

At Last

I'm determined to become friends with my G-spot. It's been this allusive thing for the bulk of my life. I didn't even know there was such a thing until college, and even then, I had no clue where mine was or what to do with it if I did find it.

✧✧✧

At the end of my marriage, my husband gives me a gift. Actually, he gives me three, but I'm not counting the two pairs of designer shoes we pick out on an evening stroll when we are trying to be kind and friendly. The gift he gives me is a "sensual awakening" ceremony. Definitely weird since the bulk of our issues pool around our sex life. I struggle to be open. My mission is to pour myself as wide open as possible, despite the fact that I am closing down to this man I'd married. He blindfolds me as I sit at the foot of the bed. The room is already dark and lit only by candles. Incense wafts in the air—thick with desire and dread. I agree to this experience despite my enormous distaste of his sexual touch because I know that if I want to shift the broken bits of me, it is best to do it when the issues arises.

He proceeds to titillate my senses. He places exotic tastes on my tongue in the form of rose, pistachio, and dulce de leche French macrons. Next, he teases my lips with cold ice cream and sticky caramel. There are things to awaken my skin—feathers, leather, and fur paddles, things to awaken my olfactory system, ylang ylang essential oil, flower petals, and things to awaken my inner ear, sensual electronic music with a hip swaying rhythm. I sit on the edge of the bed and let myself fall into this strange magical moment. All my senses are extremely heightened except for my sight. The blindfold remains wrapped around my head, allowing me to sink into the experience. I'm not sure if it is intended to be easier for me this way, but it is. I fall into the fantastical aspects of the occasion without the distraction of looking at my about-to-be-ex-husband and all the baggage his visual brings along with it.

At the time, I am reading a lot about this notion of finding God through sex. Said another way, using sex to access another plane of existence. The information I read also talks a lot about the G-spot and how it can hold sexual trauma of any kind in its cells. Lovely. Just what we don't need. A storage area for painful experiences. Wonder what the monthly rent on that is? It also said that the G-spot orgasm is more profound and deeper than a clitoral one. And that in a safe space, a partner can help release the trauma stored in the G-spot by stimulating it. They don't need to bring the woman to orgasm, rather, simply, be there as an anchor for the woman to hold on to as whatever past pain, grief, agony, rage, fear, or other trauma came up.

Still unsure about the specific details of my own childhood traumas, I know I am ready to let them go. When my about-to-be-ex-husband gently lays me down on the bed he whispers, "You're completely safe."

A silent scream screeches through my body.

Feeling my fear, he whispers, "Take a deep breath. OK. Another."

He puts his finger inside me. Breath by breath, the knots in my psyche began to loosen. His finger finds my G-spot. Breath by breath, my skin softens. His finger strokes my spot. Breath by breath, the door to my storage area opens wide. His finger prods, pulses, and pries something loose inside me. I moan, cry, scream, yelp, and utter noises I've never heard before. Grey clouds escape my pussy amidst a tumultuous sea of grief. I am a puddle when it is over. Quivering and alive. I survive the storm of my past. There is a light emerging inside me.

It's late and I'm watching *Real Sex* on HBO. There's a segment on a sex toy company that solely makes glass toys. Glass? Huh. I gawk at the toys on screen thinking, would it hurt? They seem so cold and hard, but they're pretty, smooth, and elegant looking. The company has market research testers. Yes. Real human beings whose sole purpose (at least in this TV episode) is to take glass sex toys for a spin and report on the ride. I dreamily watch the men and women out on a small yacht get jiggy with the glass objects. Seeing them moan, giggle, and play is fun. What gets me off is hearing about the toys and their purpose. The one that stops me in my tracks is the G-spot dildo. It's long, smooth, and stiff with a curved tip. Like a finger beckoning me to play.

The next day I trounce off to the Pleasure Chest. It's the longest standing erotic boutique store in Los Angeles. I was on a date ten years ago the first time I visited. It was the second date with this guy and there we were, perusing the lingerie, dildos, lotions, vibrators, nipple clamps, and other assorted sexual sundries (we ended up dating for two years). I remember hiding my nerves behind bravado and my excitement behind coolness. We purchased a few items which, opened the door to the world of sex and toys in my life.

Ten years later, alone and feeling full in my being, I walk right up to one of the sales gals, "Hi. Where are your G-spot dildos?" She takes me to a wall display filled with packaged pieces of pleasure. A slew of dildos on the left section of the wall blends into the vibrators on the right. My eyes glaze over. There's so many to look at and I'm momentarily stupefied.

"Do you have any glass ones?"

She points out the handful of them on the wall. I spot the one that looks like what I saw on TV. Being new to the whole solo exploration of the G-spot arena, I ask the sales gal about the dildo. She confirms it's the curved tip I heard about on the TV show that makes it a G-spot dildo.

And then she gives me the best advice, "Take your time to explore the G-spot. It might not happen the first time out, but when you get there it's so worth it."

I take the TV-show-looking-one off the wall. The sales gal suggests I also check out the "high end" glass toys and walks me over to a display case where they reside. I'm like a bride-to-be looking at engagement rings in Tiffany's—all atwitter and flushed. The ones in the case are so pretty. They are little, well not that little, pieces of art. Some have colored stripes, others have colored designs, and some have rhinestone and feather adornments. I suck my eyes back in my head, look at the sales gal and say, "I'll start with this one and see how we do."

As much as I enjoy masturbation, and to many people's surprise, I don't do as often as you might think. I recently had a stretch where I challenged myself to do it once a day for a week. I made it to day four. And even then, I think I fell asleep on myself. Great date huh?! It's not that I don't like to touch myself. I find my body fascinating. Alas, my body, from a young age, got keyed into having sexual pleasure with another body present. That and the fact that I grew up with a lot of visual stimulation when rubbing one out. First it was Dad's stash of Playboys in the basement. Then early morning viewings of The Benny Hill show—something about those British maids running about and cooing. Moving on to the discovery of Channel J (aka Channel 35) on New York City's fine cable network that hosted the likes of Midnight Blue with Ron Jeremy and The Robyn Bird Show (her theme song, "Baby You Can Bang My Box" still gets me wet). And yes, even the later night softcore on Showtime (back in the day when they still aired it) would do it for me. Historically, outside stimulation dictated the majority of my sexual flow. At this stage of my erotic awakening, it didn't dawn on me that there was a whole world waiting to be birthed in generating this kind of self-pleasure.

I come home with my new toy. Pretending not to notice it, I go about the usual emails and return phone calls. Later that day, putting things back in their places I unwrap the dildo. It has a red velvet pouch and a sample of lube. I'm proud of myself for purchasing it. But not enough to take it for a spin. I put it in the drawer next to the bed since it's too big for the small wooden box that holds some of the other sexual paraphernalia.

I picked up the small wooden box in Hawaii a number of years ago while on a yoga retreat. Walking through a craft fair one fine afternoon, this box grabbed my attention. It's only eight inches by four inches. Not so big that its size attracted me. The carving on the lid drew my energy to it. Taking a good look, I realized the image was of Sita and Ram—Hindu deities that had a devotional love affair. It was a signal for me to get more real about my loving. About being more aware of the big picture. I tightly wrapped the box in sarongs and then placed it in the middle of all my clothes in the suitcase for safe travels. This was the lotus seed from which I'd be reborn. Arriving home, it took me months to figure out where to put it let alone what to put in it. Ultimately, it sat empty on my nightstand.

It wasn't until I decided to experiment with using gemstones as masturbation tools that I knew what needed to live in the box. I've always been a big fan of gemstones. At first, I thought they were pretty. Then, I learned about their healing qualities. I began to gather stones. All shapes, sizes, and varieties. I had a few massage tools made out of different stones. There was a rose quartz one, a black onyx one, a purple fluorite one, and a clear quartz one. Each approximately four inches long, completely smooth, and tapered on one end. Why couldn't I use those as a dildo? This would allow me to literally take in the energy of the gemstone and access it in a more powerful way. The sacred information held within each stone could reveal itself to me. Slowly, one by one, week after week, I tried these massage tools in a way they most likely had not been intended. They were cool to the touch. A little shocking at first. The more I warmed up they did too. The rose quartz bathed my pussy in life's love. Black onyx pulled out calcified pain. Purple fluorite connected me to abundance. Clear quartz taught me bigger consciousness. These were the only stones in my "kit" at the time. I experimented with each of them, learning the nuances of the universal energy flowing between the two of us. There were many other stones out there with their own unique properties and I was eager to experience as many as possible. There was no such thing as an inanimate object.

The carved box became their home—tickling the insides, not only of me, but of Sita and Ram as well.

The days click by and the glass dildo sits in the drawer. Like Hitchcock's MacGuffins, its presence looms even when I don't see it. The irony of the situation is not lost on me. Here I am, eager, wanting, mostly aware, and in the same breath I turn my back on the thing I desire. I often wonder if this is the fate of the human condition. Desiring something and not letting ourselves receive it. This is the plight of the human mind. It is so small. And I know that if we could access all there is in the universe, we'd implode. It's too much for this dense physical existence to bear. But, getting *in touch* with the whole? Absolutely attainable.

And that's when I have the Oprah "ah-ha" moment. If I want to get to know my G-spot and all it has to offer, I must make a real date with it. I decide I'm taking myself out. Or rather, in. I prepare the surroundings. As I gather candles and incense, I feel silly. Why am I doing all this to in effect, just masturbate? Lighting a candle, the answer flickers in my consciousness—*because you are divine.* Yeah that's nice, but seriously. *Because you are important.* That voice has more oomph. It comes from a long-lost space in me and I know it's ME. The idea of treating myself as I'd like others to treat me has been simply that—an idea. Now tectonic plates grind, shift, and make their move to create new terrain in my life. Something's emerging.

I decide to take a bath. All the ancients used water ritualistically. The Mayans manipulated it to gain more power in their society.

Jewish culture performs ritual bathing for a variety of reasons. Pagans use it in most of their ceremonies to invoke specific results. Christianity uses it to baptize people. The Japanese use water rituals for many aspects of their lives. Waters all over the world have been deemed "healing" and people travel for days just to look at, soak in, or drink the magical elixir. Water's power works in two ways—it gives and it takes away. This universal wisdom carries weight. Cleansing, preparing, and honoring the body seems key for the trip I'm about to embark upon. Turning the hot water knob open all the way to the left, I smile. It's my night! The steam rises from the tap and I look into the cabinet for some bath juju. I grab a fizzy bath bomb. *Plop. Crssssss.* It dissolves releasing gold sparkles and turns the water a pinky orange. *Squirt.* A thick dollop of bath bubbles rips the water's surface sinking to the bottom. *Drip. Drip. Drip.* Three drops of Egyptian Gold essential oil gallantly dive into the water quickly filling the tub. I turn the lights off, music on, and strip the clothes from my fervent body.

The water is hot. Too hot at first. I let the cool water tap run and take my foot using it as a paddle to swish the water around the tub. When I can stand with both calves in the water without futzing about, I turn the cold water off. Slowly and surely, I slither down under the bubbles, fizz, and oil. I'm a fish marinating for dinner. Only my scales are smooth. Silky. I admire my breasts defiantly floating to the surface. I touch them. Run my palms over their surface letting my thumb and forefinger linger on the nipple. Then pinching it and pulling it towards the sky. *Mmm.* My body is coming alive.

There was a time when I hated my breasts. When I was so embarrassed by them. I was always being ridiculed because I was the girl with big boobs. Running made me look like a circus freak. Clothes either accentuated them and garnished unwanted attention or hid them making me look bulbous. All it took was that meeting with the Upper East Side plastic surgeon drawing all over me in indelible marker to change my mind about continuing to be ashamed of them or making them smaller. Call it an epiphany, God-wink, or simply a flash of personal genius but I cancelled the surgery and never looked back.

Lying in the tub, caressing my buoyed breasts—I love them. The way, when touched precisely, a shockwave of sexual arousal bolts straight to my pussy. *Wham!* It's a direct hook up. No exits on that road.

The inner soft bits of my arms find pleasure in my fingertips caress. Same with my inner thighs. Ditto with my belly. That often-chided area, the belly, becomes luscious and alive in the tub. Just as the dermal layer of my body opens from the hot water, so does my consciousness from giving myself this time. This ritual. I wonder if this loving of self will have any affect in the outer world. If I practice this enough will I become more loving? More open with a partner? More aware of my needs, desires, and wants—in and out of the bedroom? How far can this experiment go? As I wrestle with these thoughts, my fingertips officially wrinkle. Now I'm distracted. I pull the deep tub plastic suction cup doohickey off the release drain and the lever up. The tub makes its hissy gurgling noise as the water and my psycho-emotional hang ups run down the drain into the vast sewer system of the world. I hoist up and out of the tub, water glistening my candlelit skin into sparkles.

I towel off and wonder why this is such a big deal to me. How does simple pleasure become such an ordeal?

I think about a friend of mine who told me she masturbates every day. She'd sit in front of her mirror, on her bed, in the tub, on the couch, wherever she felt the mood strike her, and she'd stroke herself.

She said, "I have to give myself pleasure. Life doesn't feel right if I'm not touched regularly."

I gawked at her need for this kind of self-contemplation and her dedication to it. Honestly, a bit of it seemed rather narcissistic. The other bit seemed like she had a secret that I needed to learn. I regarded her as holding some kind of jewel that I'd never have the privilege to wear. She seemed so feminine. So aware of her womanly wiles. And in her shadow, where I often put myself, I felt downright bullish. Manly. Crude. I admired and hated her for what she wore on the surface and I was afraid to let myself exhibit the same thing. This mental separation from not only my own wholeness, but from being able to feel completely safe around her was a constant thwack in the gut. It throbbed day in and day out. This bruise reminded me how I divorced, disowned, and dislodged a major part of me. It wasn't my friend who forced the loss. She actually triggered my need to come back to claiming wholeness, not only of this feminine core but of all the pieces—wild, bold, soft, hard, sassy, demure, crass, alive. Recognizing the skewed vision of my being in the light of her forced me to not only claim all of me, but relish in all the flavors of my spectrum.

I walk into my bedroom and take a deep breath. *Here we go.* It's a cool night in Santa Monica. The windows are closed partly to keep me warm and partly to keep me protected in my own cocoon. I don't want to feel inhibited and distracted by worrying if my neighbors can hear me or me them with whatever their evening activities may be. The room smells of my favorite candle called "love." It's a mix of essential oils that the company refuses to reveal. I've enjoyed it since college, pre-candle craze, when it was only sold as an oil. It's sensual, slightly sweet, but with a bottom note that means to say, "I've got you. It's all good." I climb onto the bed, neatly made and toss the decorative pillows to the floor. The duvet cover, cool to the touch, snaps my back alive after the warmth of the bath. At first, I slip into autopilot and go straight for stimulating my clit. Going for the quick orgasm. Then I remember my intention.

Taking my hand off my pussy, I lay it on my heart and breathe. I inhale. Breath barely gets down my lungs. OK. *Deeper.* It fills my lungs. *Another.* It's moving to my sternum. *More. Take in more.* My belly rises finally pregnant with life force. *Do it again.* I do. *And again.* I do. A rhythm begins and I feel as though I'm being breathed by something else. It's my body moving but a bigger being is in the driver's seat. I open to it. There's a presence in the room. I know I'm physically alone, yet it seems like soft beings begin to emerge from the ethers. The air gets pillowy.

My skin is plumped up like there's a balloon layer between my bones and outer shell. I begin touching myself all over—elegant arms, rounded belly, juicy thighs, supple neck. The backs of my knees have new meaning as do the web-like fleshy parts between fingers. There isn't an ounce of me that's dull. Every bit is brilliant. Radiant. My whole self is a pulsing sexual open organism. Without even touching my pussy I feel it breathing. It's mouth calling and sensually yawning in pleasure. Swallowing life on new terms and spitting out the unnecessary pits.

I blindly find the glass dildo resting on the nightstand and take it in my right hand. I trace the tip down my middle from throat to Venus mound, as though I'm slicing myself bare. Resistance rests on the surface of my skin. She's crafty and seductive. Her whole tactic is to get me distracted enough from this sacred space that I fall into my old pattern of fantasize–stimulate–cum. She makes it look good as she presses with all her might to keep my pores (physical, emotional, and psychic) closed. Heavy and determined, she looks like a seasoned mixed martial arts champion ready to take home the title. I'm shy in her presence. Confrontation is not my strong suit. But that thing that breathed me, the one that took me by total surprise swoops up my flesh from the base. My belly defiantly presses into the air gulping down the new way of being. My chest bellows taking in life as throat expands singing a softly forceful moan. *You will not lure me back in.* Still holding the glass phallus, my hand moves to my pussy. The hard coolness finds my lips wanting any kind of attention. The smooth surface traces the outer lines of me and it feels mechanical. That thing bursts in and breathes me again. My belly softens and my sex widens. Wanting to go for the easy clitoral stimulation, I momentarily wrestle with the old way. The thing pushes me forward. I ease the dildo in. It's unusual and I want to reject it. A deep breath expands once again and I find hospitality for my new guest. We introduce ourselves with an in and out handshake. In and out. In and out. I realize its brash feeling is merely a guise. Like the master teachers who constantly push their disciples away with insults and ugliness only to see which ones will recognize the glory behind the harsh guts. I begin to feel the glory as the dildo wakes me up.

Being full inside my pussy is what I normally want. That sensation of having another body in me is the root claiming I long to feel. It's part of why I love to fuck. This dildo is certainly not a flesh and blood substitute, yet it's giving me a new experience. It's curved tip finds the soft fleshy mound of my G-spot sending shivers down my legs. I press into it and let the tip rub back and forth. Back and forth. I'm irritated. I'm so irritated I screech out. I feel like I'm scratching an itch that's burned, bruised, and broken. It's the kind that hurts and feels so good you don't know whether to stop or go, go, go. Tonight, I choose go. I stimulate it more. It's so annoying, painful really, that I desperately want to give up. When suddenly in a flash, I remember a past lover telling me the spot likes a windshield washer motion over it. I get a new grip on the handle and rotate the dildo side to side. *Oh*. Side to side. *Wow*. Side to side. It feels different. It feels like fingers cultivating soil making room to plant flowers. It feels ancient and good. My breath gets throaty and my spine undulates. I sense that I'm not going to be able to take this much longer. My body tightens in protest. It wants to cum. It wants the easy way out. It doesn't want to feel this much.

I pull the glass member out of my heated box.

"Uuuhhhh," escapes my mouth.

Momentary relief. Who knew masturbating could be such a chore?

Determined to stick with it I decide to let myself get into a brief stint of "easy" pleasure. My hands run over my skin, now prickly with desire. My breasts are full and are satiated with slight nipple tugs. In order to sustain the carnal joy, I take a breast in one hand, bring it to my mouth to let my tongue tease the hard tip, while the other hand strokes my velvet mound. *Oh yes*. This is where it's at. Tongue flick, finger stroke. Over and over. The muscles in my legs tighten up as does the breath in my lungs. My clit is one swollen bulge of quivering need. I can sense my fingers going into autopilot ready to launch into the quick orgasm mode. In that moment, a whoosh of consideration tackles my senses. *What are you doing?* OK. I release my breast and my pussy. That thing comes back and breathes me as I lay supine with arms at my side. Deep belly breaths. Each one reconnecting me to my original intention—find the world inside my G-spot. See what it truly has to offer.

When I land in a more centered place, I ease into continuing the task at hand while breathing open. The sheer pleasure of being full wafts over me. It's as if I've been doing it my whole life. The struggle vanished. On an out stroke, my pretend partner knocks into the spot giving me pause. It goes slower now until it decreases movement to a subtle pulse right on the spot. The joy that presses out from my insides is so intense I feel as though I'll burst into fireworks. I stay steadfast and focused on the task at hand. The goal is opening to this new layer of sex. Explore this region whose borders were closed for so long. The slight pulse shifts to a forceful repetitive tug. Not only on my G-spot, but on my breathing as well. A sound comes out of me. I'm not familiar with it. It's guttural and raw. Primal. The sound, my breath, and my body are now riding waves of pre-orgasmic pleasure. It's as if I'm cumming, but there's no tense explosion. It's more like the cum is the ocean and I'm surfing it. Dropping into the ride, my limbs sprout things that I've never seen. Starfish, gorgeous shiny flowers, planets, and tiny universes erupt from my skin. I am swollen. Everything is bigger than normal. Breath and body ride, ride, ride the surfboard of my spine.

My pussy is connected to everything. A rainbow of colors is coming in or out of her—I can't tell. Maybe it's both. The ceiling and walls of the room disappear. It's as if a smoke machine wafts pearlescent poofs of atmosphere into the air. Every single part of me begins to blend into the poofs. I'm evaporating into something larger. I feel connected to everything. In this moment, a presence, something that can only be described as a spirit, or Higher Power, floats over me. It hovers. Just long enough for me to get the concept of what's going on and then it happens. I cum and cum and cum and cum and cum and cum.

Afterwards, I'm in blissed—out shock. I lay on the bed laughing and crying. I feel bigger than ever before. I feel more profoundly connected to life. I feel—whole. Connecting with my G-spot is one of the most important things I've ever done. Does it feel a little silly? Sure. And in the same breath, no. This experience gave me a new threshold for what I'm willing to give and what I'm not willing to settle for anymore. I let the kinks smooth out. I made room for more love. I came to that thing—some people call it God.

YOUR TURN

Oneness Center

One taps into universal consciousness from this center.
True perfection, enlightenment through inner
contemplation, and unity with the omnipresent being are
all natives from this place.

Y ou are me.
   I am you.
We are all one.

Technically, we are all stardust made up of the same particles as every-thing else in the universe. And evidently, there's no separation, right?! This is the spiritual adage: We are all connected. My joy is your joy. Your pain is my pain. Their success is our success. This is what we aspire to experience. This is the kind of being-ness that could alter the world. It's the actual meaning of love thy neighbor as thyself. Mean-ing, you and your neighbor that plays music too damn loud past mid-night is you. And you're them. This is a hard pill to swallow. One that, if you swallow, can bring you unprecedented levels of peace, harmo-ny, joy, and grace on the daily. Sounds too good to be true, right?

This Oneness thing ain't for the spiritual lightweights.

   This center is here for you to get the big mamajamma course in living through your soul presence (vs. your flimsy but persistent ego personality self).

   This Oneness Center is here for your constant expansion into all that is. It is a lifelong practice and I am not sure we ever "get it" while we are still breathing. Yet, I do believe it is an endeavor worth engaging in every single day.

How are we getting there you ask?!

Why that's through your G-spot of course, she purrs.

Now, now. Before you scoff, grumble, moan, or question if the G-spot even exists, know that this is going to be a fun exploration (that's the intention for everything in this book). Let's talk a few specifics about this elusive, sought after spot.

In 1950, Dr. Ernst Gräfenberg was one of the first doctors to write about this spot in medical literature (that's why it became known as the G-spot). He described an erotic zone on the anterior wall of the vagina in close proximity to the urethra. While the G-spot and its function has continued to be a controversial topic in sexuality and science, rest assured there's *something* an inch or two inside your delicious pussy that feels different than the rest. Many people describe it as a ridged or sponge like texture. Others say that it feels a bit like tiny peas under the roof of the vagina. And some simply say, it feels a bit more lumpy than the rest. Yours may be the shy kind—smaller and tucked back. Maybe yours is a live out loud kind—distended and close to the opening of your vagina. There's no right way. There's only *your unique spot*. Remember, the possibility of erotic pleasure lives *in you*. In all your cells. They are eager to join your life's party.

Get ready to experience the delirious and delightful carnival ride that your G-spot is through these exercises and techniques.

Ready, set, let's go!

The Oneness Center—OhEmGeee! And yes, yes, yes!

Spirit Tools:

The following items can balance and invigorate the Oneness Center. Use them prior to your practice to set the tone. You increase your spiritual sexual connection by combining these spirit tools with the sex ones.

◊ Anointing with Essential Oils

This is the practice of smearing or rubbing your body with a substance to bless and consecrate your body as a sacred, energetic space. It connects the physical with the spiritual. It's most typically done with essential oils.

> **REMEMBER:** Use a carrier oil if you have sensitive skin. Almond, coconut, jojoba, olive oils are all good choices. You use a few drops of the essential oil with the carrier oil to make it easier on your skin and still reap the benefits.

Oneness Center: Dot the top, crown of your head with your index finger or both index and middle fingers. Press down on the crown with intention. You can use the palm of your hand if this feels good to *lock in* the energy of the oils.

Oils to use*:
* Olibanum (revitalizing, purifying, divine light)
* Lotus (unity with all, beauty, spiritual)
* Frankincense (holiness, calming, protective)
* Neroli (loving, peaceful, pure spirit)

◈ Elevating the Vibration with Crystals

Using crystals (forms of minerals from the earth) is as ancient of a practice as Chinese women using pearl powder for a variety of beauty benefits. Have the crystals in the room where you choose to practice, sitting next to you or placed on your body.

Crystals to use*:

- Clear Quartz (clarity, spiritual cognition)
- Diamond (invincibility, enlightenment, love)
- Herkimer Diamond (healing, enhances telepathy, purity)
- Pearl (innocence, faith, grows wisdom)

Create the Mood with Music*

You know when a certain song gets you *in the mood*. You feel lit up from the inside and all things seem—right. It's as if the world is moving exactly as it should, you are full in mind, body, and spirit. There's a flow in and around you. Consciously connect to the tunes that offer this kind of experience. You know them when you hear them.

Music to play:

- In the case of the Oneness Center, you are playing for the all and nothingness of sound. This is the kind of silence that one imagines you'd hear while floating in space. Maybe there's a distant hum. Or possibly the deep resonate OM sound from the core of the Earth? Either of these could be the soundtrack for the Oneness Center. Here, you can listen to any music that leads you to silence. Simply being in silence, sans music altogether, is also an option.

Sex Tools*:

The following items are where it's at to get your Oneness Center alive and kickin' through G-spot play. I recommend practicing with them all, but not all at once. We don't want your sweet spot to go into shock. Each tool provides a specific nuanced sensation, therefore helping you reach a new threshold in your capacity for power and pleasure.

Lube

The almighty and brilliant tool for your sexual pleasure—LUBE! It's the jelly to the nutbutter. It's the cream to your perfect latte. It's the red lipstick to your little black dress. It. Must. Not. Be. Overlooked. And I dare anyone to plead the case where lube *isn't* a good idea with penetration. We *want* you to be slippery and wet. It feels good and makes all penetration much more pleasurable. It's better for your vulvar and vaginal health too (your lady tissue is a delicate matter after all)!

As noted before, please please please be mindful of the kind of lube you use as all lubes are not made the same. We want you and your lady parts to be healthy, Mojolicious, and thriving. Choose lubes free from toxins and any chemicals that might damage your palace of pleasure and power.

G-spot Dildo and/or Vibe

Remember back from the Life Force Center section that Merriam-Webster's definition of a dildo is *an object resembling a penis used for sexual stimulation.* Just like the penis, dildos come in all shapes, sizes, colors, and materials.

For the Oneness Center, we need a *specific* dildo. One that has a curved or rounded tip. These days it's easy peasy to find them because they list them for G-spot play. My personal preference, and the one I used in the story, is the trusted glass G-spot dildo. Do not underestimate or get intimidated by its cold, hard appearance.

Sometimes the things (or even people) who have the toughest exterior are the ones that make you gush.

You may be someone that gets that extra zing from using vibrators. If so, get yourself a G-spot vibe. The bonus here is that you can use it as a dildo when the vibrating capacity it turned off and when/if you're ready for the jzzt jzzt, your toy has your back (or shall we say, spot?). So m'dear, think of a dildo or vibrator as a shaft of your choosing to worship, awaken and satisfy your Oneness Center.

Njoy Wand

This may be the holy grail for G-spot exploration with the added bonus of bringing you to ejaculate (and yes, women can ejaculate). The slang is *squirt*, but let's face it; that sounds like a sport drink. The fluid is much too sacred to be reduced to a party trick or porn fetish. Female ejaculate in the Tantric traditions is called *Amrita*, which means: nectar of the gods. That is more like it!

All Njoy products are made from high quality stainless steel. They are stunning to look at and even more so to use. Either of the wands they offer are expertly crafted to reach your peak G-spot pleasure. They didn't exist when I had my G-spot awakening, but let me say for the record, they certainly took me to higher grounds *and* gave me the capacity to ejaculate (which had never happened without the support of a lover). I swear, I'm not a spokesperson for them, but if they're reading this—call me!

Hand Towel

By this point, you know it's always a good idea to have one or more stashed nearby. This way you can luxuriate in your pleasure for as long as you like without feeling the need to get up and clean right away. Bask in your glow and enjoy!

✧ Permission:

Give it to yourself.

It's underrated and makes a world of difference.

I am giving you permission right now.

You are worthy of owning your erotic nature.

Now claim it for yourself.

Say it aloud: *I AM worthy of owning my erotic nature.*

By reading these words you are free to experiment and play with yourself, relish in your sexuality and connect it to your spiritual self. You are giving yourself a gift by doing so and therefore, you are gifting the world. When you flourish, everyone around you will as well.

SOLO PLAY:

MIND

The G-spot. Long debated. Often misconstrued. Honestly, still up for interpretation.

Yep. The G-spot has been on the hot bed of sexual education conversation for decades. She was the *it* girl in the late 80s when she first came on the scene. And everybody wanted her. But then, modern science got their paws in the mix and made it a heated debate. Is there a spot? Where is it? Does it exist? And you might be thinking all the same things.

Your invitation is to let your mind expand into new territory. The territory called, *Hello, Pussy*! That's the territory where you drop any preconceived thoughts or pent up shame and toss them out to sea for transmutation. Because here is where you get to explore something more intimate. Something expansive. Something more alluring. It's the possibility of opening to oneness. You and You. And You and everything.

You might need to let go of the idea that:

- The G-spot is a fairy tale that only exists in porn
- Orgasm through penetration is impossible
- You don't have a pleasurable spot (or spots) inside your pussy
- Only slutty women cum from this kind of stimulation
- If you don't experience pleasure from G-spot stimulation there's something wrong with you
- Or any other idea you picked up

Are you willing? Are you ready? Let's get your G on.

BODY

Like the famous line from the Vagina Monologues when asked, *If your vagina could talk, what would it say, two words?* The response: *Slooooooooow dowwwwwwwn!*

When it comes to exploring your G-spot, slow and steady is the name of the game. Your body is a sacred vessel and deserves to be treated so. Love, kindness, consideration, and collaboration get you everywhere with your body. In this specific situation, you're going for it all. You being connected to the All. It is a heady endeavor, though no need to make it precious. Your ability to connect with it all *through your all* is as accessible as ordering a latte at the local café. Yes, you need to get yourself there, request your drink order, and then wait while it's made. But it does come. And so might you.

There's a word I've come to appreciate.

Compersion.

You won't find it in the dictionary, but Wikipedia defines it as "an empathetic state of happiness and joy experienced when another individual experiences happiness and joy." Pretty cool, right?

As in, your joy is my joy. Your happiness, my happiness. Your pleasure and orgasm, my pleasure and orgasm. Oneness.

Other cultures have actual words in their dictionaries for this. In Sanskrit, *Mudita* means "the pleasure that comes from delighting in other people's well-being." In Norwegian, *Unne* means "to be happy on someone else's behalf."

Your body is an electromagnetic organism capable of sending and receiving frequency (aren't we the coolest creatures?!). When you engage in self pleasure, you can connect with the proverbial *all*. It's there for you. And that's what you're invited to experience with this Wisdom Center G-spot practice.

Claim this practice as sacred time with one, some, or all of these suggested intentions. Say them aloud with as much Mojo as you can muster.

- ✧ It is safe to explore my erotic nature
- ✧ Being erotically alive feels good
- ✧ It's good to be erotically alive
- ✧ Connecting with the universe is sexy
- ✧ I am part of the pulse of the universe
- ✧ My pussy is a portal to the sacred

✦ I love exploring new realms of pleasure in my pussy
✦ It is safe to use sex toys for exploration and awakening
✦ The more I understand the language of my pussy, the more Mojo I have

Now it's time to practice and play. Find a comfortable spot. Bed, floor, couch, or cozy chair. Whatever gives you the most joy and easy access to your pussy. In my experience, it's a good idea to have a lumbar style pillow, wedge, or regular old pillow you can fold to place under your lower back. This gives a slight tilt to your pelvic girdle and may offer easier access to your G-spot (not to mention, heightened pleasure too).

Once you're cozy and ready, cup your vulva with your palm. Wrap your hand across the naked flesh of your vulva. Say *hello, pussy*. And breathe. Nice. Slow. Deep. Breaths.

Inhale hello. Exhale fear.
Inhale yes. Exhale shame.
Inhale opening. Exhale protection.

Now, take a bit of lube and apply it on your vulva. Reconnect with her terrain. Is she feeling shy, closed up, or prudish? Or is she eager, awake, and flush? She might be somewhere in-between. It's for you to coax her alive and remind her how special she is. Use your fingers like trained vulva worshippers. How would they touch her? What feels best to her? Imagine she's guiding you with each movement. As she continues to blossom, you continue tuning into her desire. Your hand is prepping her for penetration. There's no rush. She wants you to take as much time as she needs.

There's a specific moment, a tipping point, to become intimately familiar with—it's her go signal for penetration. You might question it, or jump to it before she's ready, or hold off too long where she gets more annoyed than aroused. She doesn't give mixed messages. She is always clear. Do yourself a favor by doing your absolute best to get out of the way of her signal. When you're new to listening to her, go slow. If you think you get a signal, pause and breathe. Tune in and make sure the signal is beaming from her.

Once you have the clarity and confidence it is your Lady P speaking, she will want to pull something inside. You can tangibly feel her hunger. Her primal nature begins to purr, sigh, and ache for fulfillment.

Start with inserting one or two fingers an inch or so inside and make the *come-hither* motion. You are aiming for the anterior, belly facing wall of your pussy. Right now, you are in discovery of where and how your G-spot feels. She has a particular touch to your fingers and she generally reacts quite differently than other areas inside your pussy. Many people say the G-spot feels a bit spongy and has a ribbed like texture. See if you sense a textural shift as you slowly and gently explore.

You may feel like you have to pee when you locate the G-spot and begin to play with her. This is normal. Her structure is close to your urethra. It's a good idea to empty your bladder before engaging in this self-pleasure practice. This gives you more confidence you won't give yourself a golden shower, and allows you to relax into the pee feeling, which can ultimately result in gorgeous gushing (aka female ejaculation).

Getting back to your spot. It's critical to listen to her. She'll purr an *Oh Geeeee!* when you find her preferred pleasure. It could be through the come-hither motion. It could be from a windshield wiper motion with the pads of your fingers firmly pressed into her. It could be soft buttery strokes like a butterfly nestling on a flower stamen. Or anything else you discover.

Once you make contact, keep going. Continue using your fingers or you can introduce her to your dildo or vibrator. Using one of your toys gives you the opportunity to play with varying the depth of penetration. Remember, we're sticking close to the opening of your pussy here as opposed to going back to your crowning cervix. You are absolutely invited and encouraged to combine the two *once* you are crystal clear on how each of them feels, functions, and offers their distinct and delicious pleasure.

Experiment with rocking your hips back and forth while you have the dildo or vibrator inside. See if this motion offers an extra zing and if/when it does, pause. Do not move. Pause and breathe. You probably have been holding your breath (we all do). The key is to retrain your nervous system and neurobiological response around your pleasure from a state of fear and shut down to openness and reception. So, hang out in the bliss of the exact moment you begin to feel. The feeling may come as conventional pleasure. It may arise as slight irritation. It may annoyingly twitch like the moment before you sneeze. However, the feeling emerges, hang with it for a bit. Take a bare minimum of three slow deep belly breaths. Then, carry on. Caress, rub, tap, and groove on with your G-spot.

You will eventually find your rhythm. It's important to remember, this is *not* about having an orgasm. If it happens, cool. If it doesn't, cool. This is about widening your capacity for pleasure and deepening into your erotic nature. The more you expand in these realms, the more embodied you become. And the more embodied you become, the easier it is to transmit energy. The easier it is to transmit energy, a higher state of frequency becomes your baseline. And when a high frequency becomes your baseline, you are more connected to the One more often. This is what's possible when you awaken and enliven your G-spot.

Old emotions may arise when you activate your G-spot. Similar to the cervix, the G-spot (really all parts of your vagina) store energy. Past trauma, upsets, and abuse may come up when you expand into this realm. This is why you must be incredibly gentle with yourself. Love yourself up. Remind yourself that you are safe *right now*. You are ok. You are with *you*. What happened is not happening now. The *feelings* are there. But you are safe. You have a powerful opportunity to reprogram your body by releasing the old energy and placing new, accurate information in its place. This is why it's critical to give yourself twenty to thirty minutes for this practice. Let it be slow, luscious, and safe. Depending on where you are with your healing journey, you may need to seek counsel from a qualified trauma informed counselor*. You are your number one priority and your energetic, erotic freedom is worth moving through the tough moments.

SPIRIT*:

Sit in a quiet space where you can be undisturbed for five to fifteen minutes. Create a comfortable seat for yourself in a chair or cushion on the floor.

Light a candle if that inspires or feels good to you. A white or gold one symbolizes the Oneness Center. In addition to the candle, incorporate any of the additional spirit tools you are drawn to use for this meditation.

Gently close your eyes and begin by taking three deep breaths.
Allow your consciousness to sink into your body.
Let whatever came before this moment drift away.

Imagine you are sitting under a waterfall of white, golden light. This white, golden light is the exact right temperature. It is the perfect pressure. It is unbelievably refreshing as it cascades from above the crown of your head, down your body, across your legs and into the ground beneath you.

As the white, golden light showers down on you, it cleanses away any stress, fear, worry, doubt, or low vibration thoughts and feelings. Now, they peel and purge off you easily and readily as they are washed down into the ground beneath you to be transmuted. You allow this. With each breath you let go. And let go. And let *go*.

This white, golden light sparkles and shines washing over you. You begin to feel invigorated, alive, and sated in your own skin. Now, the white, golden light condenses above you forming a powerful column. This column focuses above your head and hovers. You begin to sense the high frequency vibration through tingling on the crown of your head. The tingling sensation urges you to mentally see the crown of your head opening, like a flower to sun. When your crown opens, the column of white, golden light easily and effortlessly begins pouring into it. It moves through your crown down into your head, then your neck, and it continues moving down the central channel of your entire body. Down through your chest, solar plexus, Life Force Center, through your root, and into the ground beneath you. You watch and feel the white, golden column dropping down, down, down deep into the Earth's core. There, it spreads out and roots in.

On an inhale, the white, golden light rises back up from the Earth's core through your root, up your Life Force Center, then solar plexus, the Heart Center, neck, head, and back up through your crown as you exhale. Now, the white, golden light rises to meet the Oneness of the universe.

On an inhale, the white, golden light descends down from the all of the universe into your crown, down through your head, neck, Heart Center, solar plexus, Life Force Center, down and out through your root as you exhale it back into the Earth's core.

You continue repeating this flow.

Inhale up from the Earth's core, exhale out the crown.

Inhale down from the universe, exhale out into the Earth's core.

Repeat for as long as you like.

Sense the white, golden light continuously moving through your central channel.

Begin to notice the moments of expansion, when you feel more full than the boundaries of your body. When the boundaries of your body begin to fade and you sense merging into All.

Imagine the dense particles of your humanness lightening up as they get infused with the white, golden light on each breath you take. Feel yourself combining with pure light. Sense your connection to the light that connects us All. Allow yourself to flow into communion with the universe.

Inhale. Exhale.

When you feel complete with your practice, finish on an inhale from your root and exhale out your crown. As you exhale this final round, see the white, golden light bursting from your crown like a dolphin spraying joyously in the ocean. Let the spray of the sparkling light twinkle down on you like fairy dust. After, resume your natural breath.

To close the practice, continue basking in the white, golden glow as you tune into the sensation of love. The kind of love that is as pure as the white, golden light. It is always around you. As you tune into this love, let it infuse every single pore and cell of your being. Let yourself get filled up by the love of the universe. Once you feel fully plumped up, shine that love light out from all your cells and pores into the universe for All. Press it out from you and share it with all living things. Feel the power of the light pressing out from you into everything in the universe.

When you are complete, seal in the practice with three deep, gorgeous belly breaths.

Slowly flutter your eyes open.

Welcome back.

* Visit *www.undressedbook.com* for your free downloadable resource lists and guided meditation

POSTSCRIPT

aka: Carry on, Pussy

We did it!
You and me.

I knew we'd get together again and I am beside myself with glee.

Being connected to you is my purpose. It gives me reason to get up every morning and carry on. I need you as much as you need me and this rejuvenated relationship is one to go out and celebrate. Not for nothing, I recommend letting all your other people with pussies know about the magic we resurrected. Cuz, hello, power to the pussy! We're better when we're *all* tapped in.

Seriously though.

Kudos to you for being the example now. We all need someone like this. Your win is a win for us all. Deborah and her pussy are super stoked they could be it for you. Oh! And they want me to remind you about an important universal law. The one of expansion and contraction. As in, it's happening all the time, every day. After taking the journey of UNDRESSED, you are probably in a state of expansion. Normal. Awesome. It's important to know you will feel a bit of contraction at some point. Normal. Also awe-some. I mean, remember, I'm the queen of expansion and contrac-tion (wink, wink). So, I got you.

The thing that makes everything smooth out is—awareness. Now that you know about the expansion, contraction gig, it won't be so alarming. Embrace them both. Like everything, there's al-ways a gem awaiting you if you're willing to receive it. I *know* you're willing. You got on board with me again! That's no small shakes.

> Please hear me say this next bit.
> In fact, let's take a deep breath.
> Inhale…
> Exhale…
> Good.
> From the bottom of me, I ask that you take this in:
> **You wear your erotic nature well.**
> And don't *ever* let anyone tell you differently.

Ok, you.

I'm forever + always,

Your Pussy 💋

EPILOGUE

I wonder where we'll be in twenty years.
I wonder what will change.
I wonder how you'll feel about your pussy then.

I deeply bow to you, the reader, for taking in the transmission of UNDRESSED.
May it bless you beyond your wildest dreams.
Spread the love + elevate the vibe.

~ Deborah Kagan
March 3, 2023
Los Angeles, CA

NOTES

Napoleon Hill, *Think and Grow Rich*

Omraam Mikhaël Aïvanhov, *Sexual Force or The Winged Dragon*

On Being podcast, Esther Perel: The Erotic is an Antidote to Death, https://onbeing.org/programs/esther-perel-the-erotic-is-an-antidote-to-death/

https://www.pennmedicine.org/news/news-blog/2018/october/inside-fear-and-its-disorders

Iris J. Stewart *Sacred Woman, Sacred Dance*

https://www.womenshealthmag.com/life/a19911220/naked-survey/

Hermes Trismegistus, *As above, so below, as within, so without...*

FURTHER RESOURCES

Deborah Kagan's Rock Your Mojo programs

You might not be ready for this journey to end. And I cannot blame you. Once you stiletto kick the door to your erotic nature and Mojo open, it tends to be only onward and upward. I say, *Yes! Yes! Yes!* You are welcome with open arms to explore any of the programs offered. They are all created keeping your expansion and evolution as a Mojoliciously alive woman top priority.

Weekly Mojo Moments delivered straight to you, free offerings, and new programs are created regularly. The best and easiest way for you to enter Mojo Central is to join the community for free. Simply go here to begin: https://mojo.deborah-kagan.com/email

UNDRESSED Resource Booklet and Guided Meditation

Visit www.undressedbook.com for your free downloadable resource booklet and guided meditation. Both of these help bring the book to new heights.

Social Connection with Yours Truly

✧ **IG:** www.instagram.com/deborahkagan
✧ **FB:** www.facebook.com/mojorecoveryspecialist

Conversations to Ignite Your Mojo

The Real Undressed podcast - https://therealundressed.com/

Books by Yours Truly

Find Your ME Spot: 52 Ways to Reclaim Your Confidence, Feel Good in Your Own Skin and Live a Turned On Life

Books by Other Mojolicious People

Existential Kink: Unmask Your Shadow and Embrace Your Power, A Method for Getting What You Want by Getting Off on What You Don't, by Carolyn Elliott PhD

The Uterine Health Companion: A Holistic Guide to Lifelong Wellness, by Eve Agee

The Seat of the Soul, by Gary Zukav

Cunt: A Declaration of Independence, by Inga Muscio

Wild Mercy: Living the Fierce and Tender Wisdom of the Women Mystics, by Mirabai Starr

Womb Wisdom Awakening the Creative and Forgotten Powers of the Feminine, by Padma Aon Prakasha

Shameless: How I Ditched the Diet, Got Naked, Found True Pleasure... and Somehow Got Home in Time To Cook Dinner, by Pamela Madsen

Polishing the Mirror: How to Live From Your Spiritual Heart, by Ram Dass

The Sweetness of Venus: A History of the Clitoris, by Sarah Chadwick

Red, Hot and Holy: A Heretic's Love Story, by Sera Beak

Women's Anatomy of Arousal, by Sheri Winston

The Apology, by V, formerly Eve Ensler

Radical Intimacy: Cultivate the Deeply Connected Relationships You Desire and Deserve, by Zoe Kors

Recommended Courses

✧ Rie Katagiri - https://www.riekatagiri.com/
Rie is the founder of Erotic Movement Arts. Brilliant, juicy offerings to keep your body and Divine Feminine alive.

✧ Ellen Heed - https://ellenheed.com/
Ellen is a seasoned somatic teacher and practitioner that helps you elegantly and powerfully awaken, heal, and transform your body

✧ Susan Bratton – https://susanbratton.com
Susan is the intimacy expert to millions and has terrific in-depth courses to expand your pleasure and sexual techniques

✦ Jules Blaine Davis - https://www.julesblainedavis.com/
Jules is The Kitchen Healer helping you to light and tend the
fire within. She's a consistent source of inspiration.

✦ Heidi Rose Robbins - https://www.heidirose.com/
Heidi is your go-to source for embodying your truest self, using the tools of astrology and poetry

Counseling and Education

✦ American Association of Sexuality Educators, Counselors and
Therapists
https://www.aasect.org/

✦ Psychology Today
https://www.psychologytoday.com

✦ Therapy Den
https://www.therapyden.com/

✦ Mental Health Match
https://mentalhealthmatch.com/

Inspiring and Important Films

What the #$! Do We (K)now!?* (2004) – directed by William
Arntz, Betty Chasse, Mark Vincente

I Am (2010) – directed by Tom Shadyac

Ask Dr. Ruth (2019) – directed by Ryan White

Becoming Nobody (2019) – directed by Jamie Catto

The Dilemma of Desire (2020) – directed by Maria Finitzo

The Business of Birth Control (2021) – directed by Abby Epstein

At Your Cervix (2023) – directed by Amy Jo Goddard

Visual Treats

✧ Alphachanneling – https://alphachanneling.com/
   The artist that brings to life the things I've felt and desire to.
   My home is full of these prints.

✧ Hannah Moghbel – https://www.instagram.com/hannahmoghbel/
   A stunning artist painting fruit and vulvas to explore ideas
   about lust, love, and feminine identity.

✧ The Vulva Gallery by Hilde Sam Atalanta – https://www.
   thevulvagallery.com/
   The much needed and glorious educational platform centered
   around illustrated vulva portraits and personal stories.

ACKNOWLEDGEMENTS

You never know when or where someone will impact your life, but when they do it's a gift.

And I am blessed with an abundance of them.

To my Mom and Dad. Thank you for being the perfect vessels bringing me back into this life and loving me through it all. Your support along this wild journey lifts my heart and is a testament to the possibility of transformation.

To D, J, M, O, S, and M. Each of you tenderized me, brought me out of slumber, and into vibrancy. I am deeply grateful.

Any ounce of success along this lengthy path to *Undressed* would not be without the support of my ladies. Thank you for being voices of reason amidst life's tornadoes. For being staunch supporters, and reminding me what I'm here to do and be. Amy Turner, Amadea Bailey, Angela Tortu, Anna Lobell, Deb Cannon, Heather Beatty, Heidi Rose, Jules Davis, Kay Richards, Khani Zulu, KJ Miller, Laurie Brucker Amerikaner, Liz Weber, Lori Snyder, Marcy Cole, Rie Katagiri, Tony Maree Torrey, and Vanessa Taal.

And to my brujas, Heather Carter, Jaqui Islas, Krystal Thompson, and Wanda Marie. Knowing you hold sacred court when called gives me great comfort. I deeply bow to you, your magical pussies, and your consistent support, not only to me, but to the Divine Feminine.

Tante E—you are the original Mojolicious woman. Your lead in life gives me courage to go for it. Thank you for the class and sass, the unwavering confidence in me, and fearlessly writing your heart out.

Eve Kagan, my sister from another mother—I bow to your dedication to healing trauma so that more of us can be free. Your eyes on early drafts of these pages invaluably transformed them. Huge gratitude for always being ready to shake your booty with me. And to be clear, you're my dance partner for life.

DJ—there is not a singular category for you, with this book or life. Your presence gives me a foundation I never knew I needed. Thank you for being unabashedly you and walking the path with me.

To Jeremy Kagan, Anneke Campbell, Alexandra Kagan, Chris Kagan, Ellen Kagan, and Mike Moynihan. Thank you for the decades of wisdom, love, celebrating life, and persevering to elevate the vibe.

I believe personal and professional success comes with greater ease when consistency and a structured group is in place. For more than seven years, that's been you, my beloved Super Group. Carlos Alvarez, David Botfeld, Demian Lichtenstein, Faith Blakeney, Josh Bolin, Keziah Dhamma, Maytal Phillips, Rachel Diamond, and Shawn Davis—thank you for holding space, calling me on my BS, reminding me of my growth, celebrating all the wins, and listening for the Deborah you know I can be.

To my weekly accountability buddy, Rachel Elise. There aren't enough words. You've been my constant for over twelve years. You've heard and seen it all. The fact that, no matter what, you continue to hold capacity for my greatness is humbling. Thank you for seeing me. Thank you for encouraging me. Thank you for never letting me give up.

This book, nor anything of substance, would see the light of day without the woman who makes all the Rock Your Mojo® programs, events, and products run smoothly for more than a decade. Judy Whitehead, you are one in a million. I thank the seemingly unfortunate way we connected—it consistently reminds me that sometimes the *bad stuff* is happening in our best interest. You continue to keep the highest interest in every woman that walks through Mojo Central. I can confidently say, we are all grateful. Thank you for your steadfast dedication and love of our women's community.

Chick—your constant Spidey-Sense and loving kicks in the ass to get me back on my path are the soul food I forget I need, but savor every time they're offered.

Anna Cherekovsky. Your hands are magic. Thank you for your healing and repeatedly midwifing my body into alignment so that my Mojo can flow.

Brian Braff and Jeff Xander. Being in front of your lens always frees me. Thank you for bringing out my true essence and capturing it for others to see. And to my girl, Martine Le Blanc. Thank you for the years of glam. No one knows how to accentuate my features and curls like you.

To Amy Freidman and Dennis Danziger for going before me and showing me the ropes.

To each of the hundreds of guests on The Real Undressed podcast—the conversations about spirit and sex keep my Mojo tank full, inspire the listeners, and peel the layers of shame off these topics. Thank you for sharing yourselves.

My team at Urano World USA. Lydia Stevens, your commitment to the spirit of this book was palpable from the start. Thank you for holding the vision with me. Your sharp editing and playful humor took the book to new heights. And to Sandra de Waard for bringing the cover design to life. You are a gem to collaborate with.

To the late great Lion himself, Peter Miller. Without you, this would not be in people's hands. Thank you for saying yes to me as a writer and fiercely advocating for this book to be in the world. I know you're out there roaring with pride.

To Charlie Serabian and Liseanne Miller for carrying the torch and amplifying its flame. Your keen support and belief in this book pushed it to the finish line.

And to my sister, Jo Moynihan. I believe a piece of Sis lives strongly in you. It is because of her I do what I do, and it is because of you I still feel unconditionally loved. YOU are the goddamn magical unicorn.

ABOUT THE AUTHOR

Deborah Kagan is a Speaker, Author, Mentor and Mojo Recovery Specialist with years of practice being a turned-on woman. She supports entrepreneurs, small business owners, consultants, creatives and the career oriented to tap into their innate power and connect with their mojo, which is a source of true self-esteem. She is the creator of the Rock Your Mojo™ programs, author of *Find Your ME Spot: 52 Ways to Reclaim Your Confidence, Feel Good in Your Own Skin and Live a Turned On Life* and hosts The Real Undressed podcast. Her methods combine over 25 years of information and experience in the fields of personal development, metaphysical studies and embodiment practices. As a philanthropist and community activist, Deborah is on the advisory board of Peace Over Violence and is the founder/executive producer of VDAY Santa Monica, a benefit raising awareness and funds to end violence against women and girls. She lives in Los Angeles. For more information, visit deborah-kagan.com.

WORKS CITED

Aïvanhov, Omraam Mikhaël. *Sexual Force or the Winged Dragon.* Pg. 35. Editions Prosveta, 5th Ed. 1997.

Aïvanhov, Omraam Mikhaël. *Sexual Force or the Winged Dragon.* Pg. 50. Editions Prosveta, 5th Ed. 1997.

Hill, Napoleon. *Think and Grow Rich.* Pg. 188. The Random House Publishing Group, 2019.

Stewart, Iris J. *Sacred Woman, Sacred Dance: Awakening Spirituality through Movement and Ritual.* Pg. 5. Inner Traditions, 2000.

Tippett, Krista, host, "Esther Perel The Erotic Is an Antidote to Death" *On Being*, 11 July, 2019. https://onbeing.org/programs/esther-perel-the-erotic-is-an-antidote-to-death/.

Winston, Sheri. *Woman's Anatomy of Arousal: Secret Maps to Buried Pleasure.* Pg. 111-112. Mango Garden Press, 2010.